THE LOST DR. BARBARA COO BEGINNERS

A Comprehensive Guide To Simple, Quick And Easy, Healthy Plant-Based Natural Recipes Inspired By Barbara O'Neill Teachings / 60-Day Meal Plan

Dr. Sofia Julius

Table of Contents

- Chapter 1 6
- THE DR. BARBARA DIET 6
- Rediscovery of Ancient Nutritional Practices 7
  - Understanding Ancient Diets 7
  - The Role of Natural Foods in Modern Health 10
- Chapter 2: Breakfasts with Historical Roots 13
  - Fermented Oat Porridge with Honey and Nuts 13
  - Herbal Infused Breakfast Scrambles 15
  - Ancient Grain Pancakes with Wild Berry Syrup 16
- Chapter 3: Revitalizing Snacks and Tonics 18
  - Dried Fruit and Nut Leather 18
  - Herbal Elixirs for Daily Vitality 19
  - Seaweed and Seed Crackers 19
- Chapter 4: Lunches from the Old World 21
  - Traditional Vegetable Stews with Bone Broth 21
  - Wild Greens and Edible Flowers Salad 21
  - Potted Shrimp with Spiced Butter 22
- Chapter 5: Forgotten Dinners 24
  - Fire-Roasted Game with Root Vegetables 24
  - Clay-Baked Fish with Herbal Stuffing 24
  - Barley and Mushroom Hot Pot 25
- Chapter 6: Ancient Sides and Ferments 27
  - Lacto-Fermented Pickles and Sauerkraut 27
  - Sprouted Legume Salad with Wild Herbs 28
- Chapter 7: Healing Soups and Broths 30
  - Medicinal Mushroom and Barley Soup 30
  - Root Vegetable and Lamb Broth 30
  - Fish Stew with Seaweed and Herbs 31
- Chapter 8: Desserts Reclaimed 33
  - Honeyed Figs with Almond Paste 33
  - Baked Quinces with Spiced Wine Reduction 33
  - Raw Carrot and Nut Cake 34

Chapter 9: Detoxifying Beverages and Herbal Teas Cleansing 35
    Cleansing Wild Berry Juice 35
    Herbal Infusion for Digestive Health 35
    Sassafras Root Beer 36

Chapter 10: Probiotic and Prebiotic Recipes from the Past 38
    Homemade Traditional Yogurt 38
    Ancient Grains Sourdough Bread 39
    Kimchi with Foraged Greens 40

Chapter 11: Plant-Based Proteins—A Historical Approach 42
    Lentil and Walnut Loaf 42
    Nettle and Pea Fritters 43
    Ancient Grain and Vegetable Patties 44

Chapter 12: Anti-Inflammatory Ancient Meals 46
    Turmeric and Ginger Stew 46
    Wild Salmon with Dill and Juniper 48

Chapter 13: Low-Glycemic Meals from Forgotten Times 50
    Roasted Turnips with Thyme 50
    Venison and Barberry Stew 50
    Pearled Barley Risotto with Wild Mushrooms 51

Chapter 14: Heart-Healthy Historical Recipes 53
    Foraged Berry Compote 53
    Grilled Trout with Wild Herbs 54
    Roasted Nuts with Sea Salt and Olive Oil 55

Chapter 15: Gluten-Free Eating from Antiquity 57
    Buckwheat Crepes with Honeyed Fruit 57
    Amaranth Pilaf with Roasted Squash 58
    Chestnut Flour Brownies 59

Chapter 16: Brain Foods from the Lost Pages 61
    Brain Foods from the Lost Pages 61
    Walnut and Pomegranate Salad 61
    Grilled Mackerel with Lemon Balm 61

Chapter 17: Beauty Recipes from Historical Traditions 63
    Beauty Recipes from Historical Traditions 63

- Cucumber and Mint Facial Mask (Edible and Topical) ... 63
- Pomegranate and Honey Scrub ... 63

Chapter 18: Family Meals from Lost Cultures ... 65
- Roast Duck with Apples and Root Vegetables ... 65

Baked Millet and Vegetables in Clay Pots ... 65

Chapter 19: Herbal Teas and Decoctions ... 67
- Wild Rosehip and Hibiscus Tea ... 67
- Dandelion and Burdock Root Brew ... 69
- Pine Needle and Citrus Tea for Immunity ... 71

Chapter 20: Seasonal Recipes ... 74
- Spring Foraged Salad with Violets and Sorrel ... 74
- Summer Fruit Tart with Ancient Grain Crust ... 75
- Autumn Root Vegetable Roast with Herbs ... 76
- Winter Squash Soup with Nutmeg and Cinnamon ... 76

Chapter 21: Special Diets from Historical Contexts ... 79
- Dairy-Free Almond Milk Pottage ... 79
- Paleo Bison Stew with Marrow Bones ... 79
- Vegan Roasted Vegetable and Nut Loaf ... 80

Chapter 22: Rediscovered Cooking Techniques ... 82
- Open Hearth Cooking Methods ... 82
- Salt Curing and Smoking of Meats ... 83

Chapter 23: Superfoods of the Ancients ... 88
- Spirulina and Barley Flatbreads ... 88
- Hemp Seed and Wild Honey Porridge ... 88
- Chia and Acai Berry Pudding ... 89

Chapter 24: Mindful Eating Practices from the Past ... 91
- Rituals Around Meals ... 91
- The Importance of Eating Seasonally and Locally ... 91
- Mindfulness in Preparation and Consumption ... 92

Chapter 25: Reconnecting With Nature Through Food ... 94
- Edible Wild Plant Identification and Use ... 94
- Creating a Kitchen Garden with Heirloom Plants ... 95
- Foraging Techniques and Seasonal Harvests ... 97

THE END 100

Copyright © 2024 By Dr. Sofia Julius

All Rights Reserved. No Part Of This Publication May Be Reproduced, Distributed, Or Transmitted In Any Form Or By Any Means, Including Photocopying, Recording, Or Other Electronic Or Mechanical Methods, Without The Prior Written Permission Of The Publisher, Except In The Case Of Brief Quotations Embodied In Critical Reviews And Certain Other Noncommercial Uses Permitted By Copyright Law.

Chapter 1

THE DR. BARBARA DIET

The Dr. Barbara Diet emphasizes a natural, plant-based approach to nutrition and wellness, inspired by the principles of Dr. Barbara O'Neill. Here are the key components of the diet:

Key Components of the Dr. Barbara Diet:

1. **Whole Foods**:
   - Focus on consuming unprocessed, whole foods.
   - Include a variety of fruits, vegetables, whole grains, nuts, and seeds.

2. **Plant-Based**:
   - Prioritize plant-based meals and minimize animal products.
   - Incorporate legumes, beans, tofu, and other plant-based proteins.

3. **Natural Ingredients**:
   - Use natural, organic ingredients whenever possible.
   - Avoid artificial additives, preservatives, and processed foods.

4. **Hydration**:
   - Drink plenty of water throughout the day.
   - Herbal teas and natural juices can also be included.

5. **Balanced Nutrition**:
   - Ensure a balance of macronutrients: carbohydrates, proteins, and fats.
   - Emphasize fiber-rich foods to aid digestion and maintain gut health.

6. **Healthy Fats**:
   - Include sources of healthy fats such as avocados, nuts, seeds, and olive oil.
   - Avoid trans fats and limit saturated fats.

7. **Sugar Reduction**:
   - Minimize the intake of refined sugars and opt for natural sweeteners like honey or maple syrup in moderation.

8. **Mindful Eating**:

- Practice mindful eating by paying attention to hunger and fullness cues.
- Eat slowly and savor each bite.

9. **Herbal and Natural Remedies**:
   - Incorporate herbal remedies and natural supplements as needed to support health.

10. **Lifestyle Integration**:
    - Complement the diet with a healthy lifestyle, including regular physical activity, adequate sleep, and stress management.

Additional Tips:

- **Seasonal Eating**: Choose seasonal fruits and vegetables to maximize nutritional value and support local farming.
- **Diverse Diet**: Include a wide variety of foods to ensure a broad spectrum of nutrients.
- **Meal Preparation**: Plan and prepare meals in advance to stay on track with the diet and avoid the temptation of processed foods.
- **Portion Control**: Pay attention to portion sizes to maintain a healthy weight and prevent overeating.

The Dr. Barbara Diet is designed to promote overall health and well-being through natural and wholesome eating habits.

Rediscovery of Ancient Nutritional Practices

Understanding Ancient Diets

Ancient diets, rooted in the traditions and wisdom of our ancestors, provide a fascinating glimpse into the culinary habits and nutritional strategies that have sustained human societies for millennia. These diets, shaped by geography, culture, and available resources, reveal a profound connection between humans and their natural environment, highlighting the intricate balance that once existed between food consumption and health.

The diets of ancient civilizations varied widely, influenced by regional climates, agricultural practices, and cultural beliefs. In ancient Egypt, for instance, the diet was predominantly plant-based, with a heavy reliance on grains such as barley and emmer wheat, which were used to make bread and beer. Vegetables like onions, garlic, and leeks were staples, and fruits such as dates and figs provided natural sweetness. Protein sources included fish from the Nile and occasional meat from domesticated animals, although meat was often reserved for the elite or for special occasions.

In the Mediterranean region, the diet of ancient Greece and Rome was rich in olives, olive oil, grains, and a variety of fruits and vegetables. Legumes, nuts, and seeds were essential components, providing necessary proteins and fats. The consumption of fish and seafood was common, given the proximity to the sea, while meat was less frequent, again reserved for the wealthy or for religious rituals. The Mediterranean diet emphasized balance and moderation, principles that continue to be recognized for their health benefits today.

The traditional diets of indigenous peoples in North and South America also offer valuable insights. Native American diets varied significantly across tribes and regions. In the Great Plains, for example, the diet was heavily based on buffalo, supplemented by wild plants and berries. In contrast, coastal tribes consumed a diet rich in fish, shellfish, seaweed, and marine mammals. The "Three Sisters" agricultural practice—growing corn, beans, and squash together—was a cornerstone of many indigenous diets, providing a balanced combination of nutrients and a sustainable farming method.

Similarly, in ancient Asia, diets were diverse and heavily influenced by local agriculture. In China, the staple foods included rice, millet, and wheat, complemented by a variety of vegetables, tofu, and fish. Tea was a significant part of daily life, both as a beverage and for its medicinal properties. In India, the diet was predominantly vegetarian, focusing on lentils, beans, rice, and an array of spices that not only enhanced flavor but also offered health benefits. The Ayurvedic dietary system, with its emphasis on balance and harmony between different body types and foods, is a testament to the sophisticated understanding of nutrition in ancient India.

These ancient diets were not only about sustenance but also about maintaining health and preventing disease. Traditional medicinal practices were often intertwined with dietary habits. For instance, in traditional Chinese medicine, food was categorized by its energy properties (yin and yang) and its ability to balance the body's internal systems. Similarly, in Ayurveda, foods were classified according to their taste, energy, and post-digestive effect, with a strong emphasis on how food impacts the body's doshas (vital energies).

One of the key lessons from ancient diets is the emphasis on whole, unprocessed foods. The absence of modern processing techniques meant that people consumed foods in their natural state, rich in nutrients and free from artificial additives. This practice inherently supported a balanced intake of macronutrients and micronutrients, contributing to overall health and well-being. Whole grains, fresh fruits and vegetables, nuts, seeds, and lean proteins provided a diverse array of vitamins, minerals, and antioxidants, essential for maintaining health and preventing chronic diseases.

The seasonal and local nature of ancient diets is another critical aspect. People consumed what was available during each season, ensuring that their diets were naturally varied and aligned with the environment. This not only supported local agriculture but also provided a range of nutrients throughout the year. Seasonal eating meant that fruits and vegetables were consumed at their peak ripeness, maximizing their nutritional value. Moreover, the local focus reduced the reliance on long-distance food transportation, promoting sustainability.

Fermentation was a common practice across many ancient cultures, used not only to preserve food but also to enhance its nutritional profile. Fermented foods like yogurt, kefir, sauerkraut, kimchi, and miso are rich in probiotics, beneficial bacteria that support gut health. The role of these fermented foods in ancient diets highlights a sophisticated understanding of the importance of gut health, long before modern science confirmed its significance.

The social and cultural dimensions of ancient diets are equally important. Food was often at the heart of community and religious practices, with meals serving as a time for gathering and celebration. Rituals and traditions surrounding food fostered a sense of belonging and continuity, reinforcing the cultural identity and passing down knowledge through generations. This communal aspect of eating contributed to mental and emotional well-being, aspects that are sometimes overlooked in modern nutrition.

In modern times, there is a growing recognition of the value of ancient dietary practices. The resurgence of interest in whole foods, plant-based diets, and traditional cooking methods reflects a desire to reconnect with the wisdom of our ancestors. Scientific research increasingly supports the health benefits of these ancient practices, linking them to lower risks of chronic diseases such as heart disease, diabetes, and certain cancers.

Furthermore, the principles of ancient diets align with contemporary concerns about sustainability and environmental impact. The emphasis on local, seasonal, and minimally processed foods reduces the carbon footprint associated with food production and transportation. This sustainable approach not only benefits individual health but also supports the health of the planet.

In conclusion, understanding ancient diets offers valuable lessons for modern nutrition. The emphasis on whole, unprocessed foods, seasonal and local eating, the inclusion of fermented foods, and the integration of dietary practices with cultural and social aspects all contribute to a holistic approach to health. By rediscovering and embracing these ancient nutritional practices, we can enhance our well-being and foster a deeper connection to the natural world.

The Role of Natural Foods in Modern Health

Natural foods, those that are minimally processed and free from artificial additives, play a crucial role in promoting health and preventing disease in the modern world. As our understanding of nutrition has evolved, the benefits of consuming natural foods have become increasingly clear, supported by a growing body of scientific evidence.

One of the primary advantages of natural foods is their rich nutrient content. Whole grains, fruits, vegetables, nuts, seeds, and lean proteins provide a wide array of essential vitamins, minerals, and antioxidants that are necessary for maintaining optimal health. These nutrients support various bodily functions, including immune response, energy production, and cellular repair. For instance, fruits and vegetables are abundant in vitamins C and A, which are vital for immune function and skin health, respectively. Whole grains are excellent sources of B vitamins, which are essential for energy metabolism.

Natural foods are also high in dietary fiber, which is crucial for digestive health. Fiber aids in the smooth movement of food through the digestive tract, preventing constipation and promoting regular bowel movements. It also plays a role in maintaining a healthy gut microbiome, the community of beneficial bacteria in the intestines. A healthy gut microbiome is linked to improved digestion, enhanced immune function, and even better mental health. Foods like fruits, vegetables, legumes, and whole grains are excellent sources of dietary fiber.

Another significant benefit of natural foods is their role in weight management. Whole, unprocessed foods tend to be lower in calories and higher in satiety compared to processed foods. They provide a sense of fullness and satisfaction, reducing the likelihood of overeating. For example, consuming a salad with a variety of vegetables, lean proteins, and healthy fats can be more satisfying and nutritious than eating a processed meal high in refined sugars and unhealthy fats. This helps in maintaining a healthy weight and reducing the risk of obesity-related diseases such as type 2 diabetes, heart disease, and certain cancers.

The antioxidants found in natural foods are powerful compounds that protect the body from oxidative stress and inflammation. Oxidative stress occurs when there is an imbalance between free radicals and antioxidants in the body, leading to cellular damage. Antioxidants neutralize free radicals, reducing the risk of chronic diseases such as heart disease, cancer, and neurodegenerative disorders. Berries, dark leafy greens, nuts, and seeds are particularly high in antioxidants, making them essential components of a healthy diet.

Natural foods also contribute to better mental health. There is a growing body of evidence linking diet to mental well-being, with natural foods playing a protective role. Nutrient-dense foods provide the brain with the necessary building blocks for neurotransmitter production and function. For example, omega-3 fatty acids found in fatty fish, flaxseeds, and walnuts are essential for brain health and have been shown to reduce symptoms of depression and anxiety. Similarly, the B vitamins in whole grains, legumes, and leafy greens are crucial for energy production and cognitive function.

The avoidance of artificial additives, preservatives, and processed ingredients in natural foods reduces the risk of adverse health effects. Many processed foods contain high levels of added sugars, unhealthy fats, and sodium, which are linked to various health issues such as obesity, hypertension, and cardiovascular disease. By choosing natural foods, individuals can reduce their intake of these harmful substances and improve their overall health. For example, consuming fresh fruits instead of sugary snacks and beverages can significantly reduce added sugar intake and the associated health risks.

Natural foods also support environmental sustainability. The production and consumption of minimally processed foods typically have a lower environmental impact compared to highly processed foods. Natural foods often require fewer resources, such as water and energy, and generate less waste and pollution. By choosing locally sourced, seasonal produce and reducing reliance on processed foods, individuals can contribute to a more sustainable food system. This not only benefits personal health but also supports the health of the planet.

Moreover, the consumption of natural foods fosters a closer connection to food sources and promotes mindful eating practices. Growing and preparing food at home encourages individuals to engage with the food they eat, understanding its origins and nutritional value. This mindful approach to eating can enhance the enjoyment of food, promote better eating habits, and reduce food waste. For example, growing a home garden or participating in a community-supported agriculture (CSA) program can provide fresh, natural produce while fostering a sense of community and environmental stewardship.

In the context of modern health challenges, such as the rise of chronic diseases and the prevalence of nutrient deficiencies, the role of natural foods is more important than ever. Incorporating a variety of natural foods into the diet can help address these issues by providing the necessary nutrients for disease prevention and overall health. For instance, the Mediterranean diet, which emphasizes natural foods such as vegetables, fruits, whole grains, nuts, and olive oil, has been associated with numerous health benefits, including reduced risks of heart disease, stroke, and certain cancers.

In conclusion, the role of natural foods in modern health cannot be overstated. Their rich nutrient content, high fiber levels, antioxidant properties, and absence of harmful additives make them essential for maintaining optimal health and preventing chronic diseases. Additionally, natural foods support environmental sustainability and promote a mindful approach to eating. By embracing the principles of natural nutrition and incorporating more whole, unprocessed foods into our diets, we can enhance our health and well-being while contributing to a healthier planet. The rediscovery and integration of ancient nutritional practices, centered on natural foods, offer a powerful strategy for addressing modern health challenges and fostering a holistic approach to wellness.

Chapter 2: Breakfasts with Historical Roots

Fermented Oat Porridge with Honey and Nuts

Fermented oat porridge with honey and nuts is a traditional breakfast with deep historical roots, cherished for its simplicity, nourishment, and health benefits. Oats, a staple grain in many ancient diets, were valued for their versatility and nutritional content. When fermented, oats undergo a natural process that enhances their digestibility and nutrient absorption, making them easier on the digestive system.

To prepare fermented oat porridge, whole oats are soaked in water and sometimes a fermenting agent like yogurt or kefir for several hours or overnight. This soaking period allows beneficial enzymes to break down complex carbohydrates and reduce phytic acid, enhancing nutrient bioavailability. Fermentation also promotes the growth of beneficial bacteria, similar to those found in probiotic-rich foods, which can support gut health and digestion.

After soaking, the oats are cooked gently with water or milk until they reach a creamy consistency. The addition of honey provides natural sweetness and additional nutrients, while nuts such as almonds, walnuts, or pecans add texture, protein, and healthy fats. This combination not only satisfies hunger but also provides sustained energy throughout the morning, making it an ideal choice for starting the day.

Historically, fermented oat porridge was a common breakfast across many cultures. In Scandinavian countries, for example, fermented oat porridge known as "sour porridge" or "sour gruel" was a traditional dish, often enjoyed with berries, honey, or dried fruits. It was valued for its ability to sustain energy levels during long, cold winters and provide essential nutrients for physical labor.

In ancient Greece and Rome, porridge made from various grains, including oats, was a staple breakfast food. It was typically cooked with water or milk and flavored with honey, nuts, or fruits. This simple yet nutritious meal provided energy for daily activities and was often eaten alongside bread and olives.

Today, fermented oat porridge continues to be appreciated for its health benefits and comforting qualities. It serves as a canvas for creativity, allowing individuals to customize their breakfast with different toppings such as fresh fruits, seeds, or spices. The incorporation of fermented foods into breakfast not only enhances flavor but also supports digestive health and overall well-being.

Herbal Infused Breakfast Scrambles

Herbal infused breakfast scrambles offer a flavorful and nutritious twist on traditional scrambled eggs, incorporating a variety of fresh herbs and vegetables for added taste and health benefits. Scrambled eggs have a long history as a popular breakfast dish, valued for their protein content and versatility in culinary traditions worldwide. By infusing them with herbs, this dish not only enhances flavor but also introduces additional nutrients and medicinal properties.

To prepare herbal infused breakfast scrambles, start by whisking eggs with a splash of milk or cream until well combined. Fresh herbs such as parsley, chives, basil, or cilantro are finely chopped and added to the egg mixture, along with diced vegetables like tomatoes, spinach, bell peppers, or mushrooms. Herbs not only contribute aromatic flavors but also provide essential vitamins, minerals, and antioxidants that support overall health.

In ancient Rome, eggs were a common breakfast food, often prepared in various ways including scrambled with herbs and vegetables. The addition of herbs such as coriander and parsley added depth of flavor while providing medicinal benefits. In medieval Europe, scrambled eggs were enjoyed by nobility and commoners alike, often seasoned with herbs and spices from the garden.

The modern interpretation of herbal infused breakfast scrambles aligns with contemporary preferences for fresh, seasonal ingredients and nutritious meals. Herbs are known for their antioxidant properties, which help combat oxidative stress and inflammation in the body. They also contain essential oils and phytonutrients that support immune function and overall well-being.

By incorporating a variety of herbs into breakfast scrambles, individuals can enjoy a flavorful dish that promotes health and vitality. Fresh herbs can be grown at home or sourced from local farmers' markets, ensuring quality and freshness. Experimenting with different herb combinations allows for culinary creativity while maximizing nutritional benefits.

Ancient Grain Pancakes with Wild Berry Syrup

Ancient grain pancakes with wild berry syrup combine the wholesome goodness of ancient grains with the vibrant flavors of seasonal berries, offering a nutritious and satisfying breakfast option with historical roots. Ancient grains, such as spelt, einkorn, or teff, have been cultivated for thousands of years and valued for their nutritional density and resilience in diverse growing conditions.

To prepare ancient grain pancakes, a blend of ancient grain flour—often a mix of different grains—is combined with baking powder, salt, and a sweetener such as honey or maple syrup. Eggs, milk or a plant-based alternative, and melted butter or oil are added to create a smooth batter. This batter is then cooked on a hot griddle until golden brown and fluffy.

Wild berry syrup, made from fresh or frozen berries such as strawberries, blueberries, raspberries, or blackberries, adds a burst of natural sweetness and antioxidants. Berries are simmered with a small amount of water and a sweetener like honey or agave nectar until they break down into a thick, flavorful syrup. This colorful and nutrient-rich topping enhances the taste of pancakes while providing vitamins, minerals, and phytonutrients.

Throughout history, pancakes made from grains and cereals have been enjoyed across cultures as a comforting and nourishing breakfast food. In ancient Greece and Rome, pancakes made from wheat flour were a popular choice, often served with honey or fruit preserves. In medieval Europe, pancakes were made from a variety of grains, including barley, oats, and rye, and cooked over an open fire or on a griddle.

Today, ancient grain pancakes with wild berry syrup appeal to contemporary tastes for wholesome and nutritious breakfast options. Ancient grains are recognized for their high fiber content, which supports digestive health and helps regulate blood sugar levels. They also contain essential vitamins and minerals, such as iron, magnesium, and B vitamins, which are important for energy production and overall well-being.

The inclusion of wild berries in the syrup provides a rich source of antioxidants, which help protect cells from oxidative damage and promote cardiovascular health. Berries are also low in calories and rich in dietary fiber, making them a healthy addition to pancakes without compromising flavor or nutrition.

By incorporating ancient grain pancakes with wild berry syrup into their breakfast routine, individuals can enjoy a delicious and nutrient-dense meal that honors historical culinary traditions while supporting modern health goals. This wholesome breakfast option provides sustained energy, promotes digestive health, and delivers essential nutrients, making it a satisfying choice for starting the day on a nourishing note.

Chapter 3: Revitalizing Snacks and Tonics

Dried Fruit and Nut Leather

Dried fruit and nut leather, a traditional snack with roots in ancient preservation techniques, offers a revitalizing combination of natural sweetness, nutrients, and energy. This snack, also known as fruit leather or fruit roll-up, has been enjoyed across cultures for centuries as a convenient and nutritious way to preserve fruits and nuts for extended periods.

To prepare dried fruit and nut leather, fresh fruits such as apples, apricots, figs, or berries are pureed into a smooth consistency. Nuts like almonds, walnuts, or cashews are finely chopped or ground into a meal. The fruit puree is combined with the nut meal, along with honey or another natural sweetener, and spread thinly onto a baking sheet or parchment paper. It is then dried slowly in a low-temperature oven or dehydrator until it becomes leathery and pliable.

Historically, dried fruit and nut leather served as a portable and long-lasting food source, ideal for travelers, explorers, and nomadic societies. In ancient Mesopotamia, dried fruits such as dates and figs were prized for their energy-boosting properties and ability to withstand harsh climates. The addition of nuts provided essential fats, proteins, and additional nutrients, making this snack a valuable source of sustenance.

In medieval Europe, dried fruit and nut combinations were popular among nobility and commoners alike, often enjoyed during long journeys or as a nutritious addition to meals. The drying process not only preserved the fruits and nuts but also concentrated their flavors and nutrients, making them a flavorful and satisfying snack.

Today, dried fruit and nut leather continues to be appreciated for its convenience, flavor, and health benefits. It serves as a wholesome alternative to processed snacks high in sugars and artificial additives. The combination of fruits and nuts provides a balanced source of carbohydrates, proteins, healthy fats, vitamins, and minerals, making it an ideal choice for a quick energy boost or post-workout recovery.

Herbal Elixirs for Daily Vitality

Herbal elixirs for daily vitality offer a rejuvenating blend of herbs, spices, and natural ingredients designed to support overall health and well-being. Elixirs have a long history dating back to ancient civilizations, where medicinal plants and herbal remedies were valued for their therapeutic properties and ability to promote vitality.

To prepare herbal elixirs, a combination of fresh or dried herbs such as ginger, turmeric, mint, or elderflower is steeped in hot water to extract their beneficial compounds. Additional ingredients like honey, lemon juice, or apple cider vinegar may be added to enhance flavor and provide additional health benefits. The resulting infusion is strained and consumed as a warm or chilled beverage, depending on personal preference.

In ancient Egypt, herbal elixirs made from medicinal plants such as hibiscus, chamomile, and licorice root were revered for their healing properties and ability to promote longevity. These elixirs were often consumed daily as part of a holistic approach to health and well-being, supporting digestive health, immune function, and mental clarity.

Similarly, in traditional Chinese medicine, herbal teas and elixirs have been used for centuries to balance the body's energy systems (Qi) and support vital organs such as the liver, kidneys, and heart. Ingredients like ginseng, astragalus, and goji berries were commonly included in elixirs to enhance vitality, strengthen immunity, and promote longevity.

Today, herbal elixirs continue to be valued for their therapeutic benefits and natural approach to wellness. They serve as a refreshing alternative to sugary beverages and caffeinated drinks, offering hydration along with a variety of health-promoting compounds. The versatility of herbal elixirs allows for customization based on individual health goals and preferences, whether for relaxation, energy boost, or immune support.

Seaweed and Seed Crackers

Seaweed and seed crackers provide a nutritious and revitalizing snack option that combines the natural flavors and benefits of seaweed with the crunch of seeds and whole grains. Seaweed, rich in minerals such as iodine, calcium, and magnesium, offers numerous health benefits and has been a staple in coastal diets for centuries.

To prepare seaweed and seed crackers, a mixture of whole grains, seeds such as sesame, chia, or pumpkin seeds, and dried seaweed flakes or powder is combined with water and olive oil to form a dough. The dough is rolled out thinly and cut into individual crackers, which are baked until crisp and golden brown. The addition of sea salt or herbs enhances flavor while providing additional nutrients.

Historically, seaweed was valued for its nutritional density and availability along coastal regions. In ancient Japan, seaweed such as nori, wakame, and kombu was a fundamental part of the diet, providing essential minerals and vitamins. Seaweed was often dried and preserved for long-term storage, making it a valuable source of sustenance during lean times.

In medieval Europe, seaweed was used in culinary practices and herbal remedies for its medicinal properties and rich nutrient content. Seaweed crackers and biscuits were enjoyed by sailors and explorers as a portable and nutrient-dense snack during long sea voyages.

Today, seaweed and seed crackers continue to gain popularity as a nutritious and flavorful snack option. They are appreciated for their crunchy texture, savory flavor, and high nutritional value. Seaweed provides essential minerals that support thyroid function, bone health, and overall vitality. Seeds contribute healthy fats, proteins, and fiber, promoting satiety and supporting digestive health.

By incorporating seaweed and seed crackers into the diet, individuals can enjoy a satisfying snack that offers a unique combination of flavors and nutrients. These crackers are a wholesome alternative to traditional processed snacks, offering essential vitamins, minerals, and antioxidants that promote health and well-being. Whether enjoyed on their own or paired with dips or spreads, seaweed and seed crackers provide a revitalizing snack option that honors culinary traditions while supporting modern dietary preferences.

Chapter 4: Lunches from the Old World

Traditional Vegetable Stews with Bone Broth

Traditional vegetable stews with bone broth are a hallmark of many old-world cuisines, celebrated for their nourishing properties and deep, comforting flavors. Across various cultures, from European to Middle Eastern, these stews often feature a robust base of bone broth—a nutrient-dense liquid made by simmering bones in water with aromatics and herbs. The slow-cooking process extracts gelatin, collagen, and essential minerals from the bones, enriching the broth with health-promoting benefits.

In Mediterranean traditions, such as Italian minestrone or French pot-au-feu, vegetable stews are crafted with seasonal produce, ensuring both freshness and flavor. Root vegetables like carrots and parsnips add sweetness, while leafy greens such as kale or spinach provide vibrant color and essential nutrients. The addition of bone broth not only enhances the stew's richness but also supports joint health and digestion due to its collagen content.

Across Eastern European cuisines, hearty vegetable and cabbage stews like Russian borscht or Polish kapusniak showcase a fusion of local ingredients and centuries-old culinary techniques. These dishes often incorporate fermented elements like sauerkraut or sour cream, which contribute probiotics for gut health alongside the stew's hearty warmth.

In the Middle East, dishes like Moroccan tagine or Persian khoresh combine vegetables with aromatic spices such as cumin, turmeric, and cinnamon, creating a sensory journey through layers of flavor. Bone broth in these stews serves not only as a base but also as a symbol of hospitality and nourishment deeply embedded in cultural practices.

Wild Greens and Edible Flowers Salad

Wild greens and edible flowers salads evoke a connection to nature and a celebration of seasonal abundance, offering a refreshing contrast to heartier dishes commonly found in old-world cuisine. Across various regions, from the Mediterranean to Scandinavia, these salads showcase a tapestry of flavors and textures, often foraged or sourced locally.

In Mediterranean diets, salads featuring wild greens like dandelion, arugula, or purslane are staples, rich in vitamins, minerals, and antioxidants. Paired with edible flowers such as nasturtiums or violets, these salads not only provide a burst of color but also offer unique flavor profiles—from peppery to subtly sweet—that elevate the dining experience.

In Northern European traditions, salads composed of foraged greens like nettle or sorrel reflect a deep connection to the land and a reverence for seasonal eating. These greens, often rich in iron and vitamins, are tenderly dressed with simple vinaigrettes or herb-infused oils, preserving their natural essence while complementing the flavors of the accompanying dishes.

In the Middle East, salads featuring wild herbs like mint, parsley, and purslane are commonplace, offering a refreshing counterpart to spiced meats and grain-based dishes. Edible flowers such as rose petals or borage add a delicate touch, symbolizing prosperity and beauty in culinary traditions.

Potted Shrimp with Spiced Butter

Potted shrimp with spiced butter epitomizes the indulgent simplicity of old-world seafood dishes, celebrated for their rich flavors and historical significance. Originating from coastal regions across Europe, these dishes showcase a meticulous preparation process that preserves the delicate essence of shrimp while enhancing it with aromatic spices and clarified butter.

In British cuisine, potted shrimp—a beloved delicacy since the Victorian era—is prepared by gently simmering fresh shrimp in seasoned butter, often infused with mace, nutmeg, and lemon zest. The slow cooking process allows the flavors to meld, creating a luxurious spread that is traditionally enjoyed with crusty bread or toast points.

Across the Channel, French variations like crevettes grises au beurre d'épices feature small gray shrimp delicately poached in a fragrant blend of butter and herbs, such as tarragon and chervil. These preparations highlight the artisanal craftsmanship of French gastronomy, where attention to detail and quality of ingredients are paramount.

In Scandinavian traditions, potted shrimp dishes such as räkmacka showcase a fusion of local seafood with globally inspired spices, often incorporating elements like dill, horseradish, and mustard seeds. These combinations not only reflect the region's maritime heritage but also exemplify its commitment to sustainable fishing practices and culinary innovation.

Lunches from the Old World offer a glimpse into culinary traditions shaped by centuries of cultural exchange and regional diversity. Whether through hearty stews simmered in bone broth, vibrant salads adorned with wild greens and edible flowers, or indulgent seafood dishes like potted shrimp with spiced butter, these meals encapsulate more than just sustenance—they embody a shared heritage of craftsmanship, nourishment, and the timeless art of gathering around the table.

Chapter 5: Forgotten Dinners

Fire-Roasted Game with Root Vegetables

Fire-roasted game with root vegetables harkens back to ancient culinary traditions where cooking over an open flame was both a necessity and an art form. Across cultures and continents, from North America to Europe and beyond, this method of preparing wild game—such as venison, wild boar, or game birds—has been integral to sustaining communities and celebrating regional flavors.

In North American Indigenous cultures, game roasting techniques varied widely but often involved slow cooking meats like bison or elk over open flames or hot stones. Accompanying root vegetables such as potatoes, carrots, and turnips were wrapped in leaves or clay, infusing them with smoky flavors and preserving their natural sweetness.

European traditions of fire-roasted game often centered around communal feasts and seasonal hunting rituals. Dishes like French roti de cerf (roast venison) or Scottish roast grouse showcased local game meats seasoned with aromatic herbs like thyme, rosemary, and juniper berries. Root vegetables, roasted alongside the game, provided sustenance and a rustic complement to the rich flavors of the meat.

In Scandinavian cultures, fire-roasted game such as reindeer or wild fowl was prepared during winter hunts and festivities. The use of juniper branches or wood chips imparted a distinct smokiness to the meats, while root vegetables like parsnips and rutabagas added earthy notes, creating a balanced and hearty meal cherished in Nordic culinary heritage.

Clay-Baked Fish with Herbal Stuffing

Clay-baked fish with herbal stuffing represents a time-honored technique where fish, often freshly caught from nearby waters, is encased in clay and baked over open coals or in traditional clay ovens. This method, prevalent in coastal regions worldwide, preserves the fish's moisture while infusing it with the aromatic essence of herbs and spices.

Mediterranean cultures have long practiced clay-baked fish dishes such as Greek psaristokastano (fish baked in clay) or Spanish pescado al horno de arcilla, where whole fish like sea bass or red snapper are stuffed with fresh herbs such as parsley, dill, and oregano before being encased in clay. This process seals in flavors and juices, resulting in tender, succulent fish that remains moist and flavorful.

In South American traditions, clay-baked fish preparations like Peruvian pescado al hornoenarcilla emphasize local ingredients such as cilantro, aji amarillo peppers, and native herbs. Wrapped in banana leaves before being covered in clay, these dishes exemplify a fusion of ancient cooking methods with vibrant regional flavors, creating a culinary experience that honors both tradition and innovation.

Asian cuisines, particularly in Southeast Asia, feature clay-baked fish dishes such as Thai pla pao (salt-crusted grilled fish) or Indonesian ikan panggang. These preparations often include a blend of aromatic herbs like lemongrass, kaffir lime leaves, and galangal, which impart complex flavors to the fish while preserving its natural texture and moisture.

Barley and Mushroom Hot Pot

Barley and mushroom hot pot exemplifies the hearty simplicity of forgotten dinners, where humble ingredients are transformed into nourishing meals that warm the body and soul. Across agricultural societies, from Europe to East Asia, barley—a versatile grain rich in fiber and nutrients—has been a staple in traditional diets, often combined with seasonal mushrooms to create satisfying one-pot dishes.

In European peasant cuisines, barley and mushroom hot pots like Scottish Scotch broth or Russian shchi showcased the resourcefulness of rural communities, utilizing locally grown barley and foraged mushrooms to create robust soups or stews. Slow simmering allowed the flavors to meld, producing dishes that offered sustenance during long winters and seasonal hardships.

In East Asian traditions, barley and mushroom hot pots such as Japanese shimeji nabemono or Korean boribap highlighted the region's affinity for communal dining and seasonal ingredients. Barley, often soaked or parboiled before cooking, provided a nutty undertone to the dish, while mushrooms like shiitake or enoki added umami richness, enhancing the overall depth of flavor.

Across the Middle East and North Africa, barley and mushroom hot pots such as Moroccan harira or Iranian ash-e-jow often incorporated a blend of spices and herbs like cinnamon, cumin, and mint, transforming simple ingredients into aromatic and hearty soups that nourished both body and spirit.

Forgotten dinners offer a glimpse into culinary traditions shaped by resilience, resourcefulness, and a deep connection to the land. Whether through fire-roasted game with root vegetables, clay-baked fish with herbal stuffing, or barley and mushroom hot pot, these dishes embody more than just sustenance—they reflect a shared heritage of ingenuity, sustainability, and the enduring art of creating meals that unite communities across time and place.

Chapter 6: Ancient Sides and Ferments

Lacto-Fermented Pickles and Sauerkraut

Lacto-fermented pickles and sauerkraut are time-honored preservation techniques that have been cherished for centuries across cultures worldwide. Rooted in the necessity of preserving seasonal produce, these fermented foods not only extend shelf life but also enhance nutritional value and flavor, making them staples in ancient culinary traditions.

In Eastern European cuisines, sauerkraut—a fermented cabbage dish—has been a cornerstone of winter diets for centuries. Prepared by layering shredded cabbage with salt and allowing natural bacteria to ferment it over several weeks, sauerkraut develops a tangy flavor and crunchy texture. Rich in probiotics and vitamin C, sauerkraut not only aids digestion but also boosts immune health, making it a valuable addition to traditional dishes like German bratwurst or Polish pierogi.

Across Asia, lacto-fermented pickles such as Korean kimchi or Japanese tsukemono reflect regional flavors and seasonal ingredients. Kimchi, made from fermented vegetables like Napa cabbage and radishes seasoned with garlic, ginger, and chili pepper, undergoes a transformative fermentation process that enhances its probiotic content and umami flavor profile. Tsukemono, on the other hand, encompasses a variety of pickled vegetables like cucumbers and daikon radishes, offering a refreshing accompaniment to rice-based meals and sushi.

In the Middle East and Mediterranean regions, lacto-fermented vegetables such as Lebanese pickled turnips or Turkish torshi demonstrate a culinary artistry that balances tanginess with herbal aromatics. These pickles, often preserved in brine with spices like coriander seeds and peppercorns, add brightness and depth to mezze platters and grilled meats, showcasing a cultural appreciation for bold flavors and preservation techniques.

Spiced Apple Chutney

Spiced apple chutney epitomizes the art of preserving fruits with aromatic spices and vinegar—a tradition steeped in British colonial history and Indian culinary influence.

Originating from the word "chatni" in Hindi, meaning to lick or taste, chutneys were originally crafted to accompany rice, breads, and meats, offering a balance of sweet, sour, and savory flavors.

In British cuisine, spiced apple chutney emerged as a way to utilize abundant apple harvests and preserve them for year-round enjoyment. Simmered with onions, vinegar, brown sugar, and a medley of spices like cinnamon, cloves, and ginger, apple chutney develops a complex flavor profile that enhances everything from cheese platters to roasted meats. The slow cooking process allows the flavors to meld, resulting in a condiment that balances sweetness with a hint of tanginess—a hallmark of traditional British preserves.

In Indian gastronomy, chutneys like mango or tamarind have been integral to regional cuisines for centuries, providing a burst of flavor alongside spicy curries and aromatic rice dishes. Spiced apple chutney, with its adaptation of local ingredients and spices, exemplifies the fusion of British and Indian culinary traditions, showcasing a versatility that extends beyond traditional boundaries.

Sprouted Legume Salad with Wild Herbs

Sprouted legume salad with wild herbs celebrates the nutritional bounty of sprouted seeds and foraged greens—a practice dating back to ancient civilizations that recognized the health benefits of germinating seeds and incorporating wild plants into daily diets. Sprouting enhances the bioavailability of nutrients and enzymes, making legumes easier to digest while preserving their nutritional integrity.

In Mediterranean diets, salads featuring sprouted legumes like chickpeas or lentils are often paired with wild herbs such as purslane, dandelion greens, and wild fennel. These greens, rich in vitamins and antioxidants, add a fresh, earthy dimension to the salad while promoting digestive health and supporting overall wellness. Drizzled with olive oil and lemon juice, sprouted legume salads exemplify a commitment to seasonal eating and sustainable agriculture.

In Native American cultures, sprouted legumes such as beans or corn were traditionally combined with wild herbs like lamb's quarters or amaranth, creating nutrient-dense salads that sustained communities through harsh winters and seasonal migrations. These salads not only provided essential vitamins and minerals but also honored a deep connection to the land and its natural resources.

In East Asian traditions, sprouted legume salads like mung bean or adzuki bean sprouts are seasoned with sesame oil, soy sauce, and toasted sesame seeds, reflecting a harmony of flavors and textures that enhance the salads' nutritional value. Wild herbs such as watercress or mustard greens add a peppery note, balancing the dish with a subtle complexity that complements rice-based meals and grilled proteins.

Ancient sides and ferments offer a journey through time, revealing culinary practices that prioritize preservation, flavor enhancement, and nutritional richness. Whether through lacto-fermented pickles and sauerkraut, spiced apple chutney, or sprouted legume salad with wild herbs, these dishes embody the ingenuity of ancient civilizations in harnessing the natural bounty of the earth to create nourishing accompaniments that enrich meals and traditions alike.

Chapter 7: Healing Soups and Broths

Medicinal Mushroom and Barley Soup

Medicinal mushroom and barley soup combines the earthy richness of mushrooms with the hearty texture of barley, creating a comforting and nourishing dish. This soup not only satisfies the palate but also offers numerous health benefits, thanks to its key ingredients.

Mushrooms, especially varieties like shiitake, maitake, and reishi, are known for their immune-boosting properties. They contain polysaccharides and beta-glucans that support the immune system by enhancing its response to infections and inflammation. Additionally, mushrooms are rich in antioxidants, which help combat oxidative stress and reduce the risk of chronic diseases.

Barley, a versatile grain, adds a chewy texture to the soup while contributing significant nutritional benefits. It is a good source of dietary fiber, which promotes digestive health and helps regulate blood sugar levels. Barley also contains essential minerals such as manganese, selenium, and phosphorus, which are vital for overall health.

The combination of mushrooms and barley in this soup creates a synergistic effect, providing a robust nutritional profile that supports immunity, digestion, and overall well-being. When preparing this soup, simmering the ingredients allows their flavors to meld together, resulting in a savory broth that warms both the body and soul.

Root Vegetable and Lamb Broth

Root vegetable and lamb broth is a hearty and nutrient-rich soup that combines the sweetness of root vegetables with the savory richness of lamb. This traditional dish not only offers comfort but also delivers essential vitamins, minerals, and proteins necessary for optimal health.

Root vegetables such as carrots, parsnips, and turnips are packed with vitamins (like vitamin A, C, and K) and minerals (such as potassium and magnesium) that support various bodily functions. They are also high in dietary fiber, promoting digestive health and helping maintain a healthy weight.

Lamb, a flavorful and tender meat, provides high-quality protein along with essential nutrients like iron, zinc, and B vitamins. These nutrients are crucial for muscle growth, immune function, and energy production. When simmered in broth, lamb adds depth to the flavor profile while infusing the soup with its nutritional benefits.

The slow simmering process of this broth allows the flavors of the root vegetables and lamb to meld together, creating a rich and satisfying soup that is both nourishing and comforting. Whether enjoyed as a starter or a complete meal, root vegetable and lamb broth provides a wholesome dining experience that promotes overall well-being.

Fish Stew with Seaweed and Herbs

Fish stew with seaweed and herbs combines the delicate flavors of seafood with the umami richness of seaweed, enhanced by aromatic herbs. This dish not only tantalizes the taste buds but also offers a plethora of health benefits, making it a popular choice for both culinary enjoyment and nutritional value.

Fish, particularly varieties like salmon, cod, or halibut, is rich in omega-3 fatty acids, which are essential for heart health, brain function, and reducing inflammation. Omega-3s also support skin health and may reduce the risk of chronic diseases such as heart disease and arthritis.

Seaweed, often considered a superfood, adds depth to the stew with its unique flavor profile and impressive nutrient content. It is an excellent source of iodine, essential for thyroid function, and contains vitamins (such as vitamin K and folate) and minerals (like calcium and magnesium) that support overall health.

Herbs like thyme, parsley, and dill not only enhance the flavor of the stew but also contribute antioxidants and other bioactive compounds that promote health and well-being. These herbs provide anti-inflammatory and antimicrobial properties, supporting immune function and aiding in digestion.

The combination of fish, seaweed, and herbs in this stew creates a harmonious blend of flavors and nutrients that nourish the body and satisfy the senses. Whether enjoyed as a light meal or a comforting dinner option, fish stew with seaweed and herbs offers a delicious way to incorporate seafood and nutrient-dense ingredients into your diet.

Each of these soups and broths exemplifies the principles of healing through food, offering both nourishment and therapeutic benefits. Whether you're seeking immune support, digestive health, or simply a comforting meal, these recipes provide a delicious way to promote overall well-being.

Chapter 8: Desserts Reclaimed

Honeyed Figs with Almond Paste

Honeyed figs with almond paste offer a delightful combination of sweet, fruity flavors and nutty richness. This dessert not only satisfies the craving for something sweet but also provides a range of nutritional benefits from its wholesome ingredients.

Figs, a naturally sweet fruit, are rich in dietary fiber, potassium, and antioxidants such as flavonoids and polyphenols. These nutrients contribute to digestive health, support heart function, and help reduce oxidative stress in the body. Figs also provide natural sugars that satisfy the sweet tooth without causing a rapid spike in blood sugar levels.

Almond paste, made from ground almonds and sweetened with honey or sugar, adds a creamy and nutty element to the dessert. Almonds are packed with healthy fats, protein, fiber, and essential vitamins and minerals like vitamin E, magnesium, and calcium. They promote heart health, aid in weight management, and support bone strength.

The combination of honeyed figs and almond paste creates a decadent yet nutritious dessert that can be enjoyed on its own or paired with a variety of accompaniments such as yogurt or a drizzle of honey. This dessert celebrates the natural sweetness of figs while incorporating the nourishing benefits of almonds, making it a satisfying and wholesome choice.

Baked Quinces with Spiced Wine Reduction

Baked quinces with spiced wine reduction offer a sophisticated dessert experience that combines the delicate sweetness of quinces with the aromatic richness of spiced wine. This dessert not only delights the senses but also provides a range of health benefits from its unique ingredients.

Quinces, a relative of apples and pears, offer a fragrant and slightly tart flavor when baked. They are rich in dietary fiber, vitamins (such as vitamin C and B-complex vitamins), and minerals (including potassium and copper). Quinces support digestive health, immune function, and help regulate blood pressure.

Spiced wine reduction, infused with warming spices like cinnamon, cloves, and star anise, enhances the flavor profile of the dessert while providing antioxidant properties. These spices have anti-inflammatory effects and may help improve circulation and digestion.

Together, baked quinces and spiced wine reduction create a luxurious dessert that showcases the natural flavors of seasonal fruit and the aromatic complexity of spices. Whether served warm with a dollop of whipped cream or enjoyed cold with a scoop of ice cream, this dessert offers a sophisticated way to indulge in the natural goodness of quinces and spices.

Raw Carrot and Nut Cake

Raw carrot and nut cake is a wholesome dessert option that combines the sweetness of carrots with the richness of nuts and dried fruits, offering a nutritious alternative to traditional cakes. This dessert not only satisfies the sweet tooth but also provides a range of health benefits from its nutrient-dense ingredients.

Carrots, known for their vibrant color and sweet flavor, are rich in beta-carotene (a precursor to vitamin A), fiber, and antioxidants. These nutrients support eye health, immune function, and promote healthy skin. Carrots also provide natural sweetness, making them a perfect ingredient for healthier dessert options.

The nut and dried fruit base of the cake typically includes ingredients like almonds, walnuts, dates, and raisins. Nuts are excellent sources of healthy fats, protein, and essential minerals such as magnesium and phosphorus. They support heart health, aid in weight management, and provide sustained energy.

The combination of carrots, nuts, and dried fruits in this cake offers a satisfying texture and flavor profile that appeals to both adults and children. Whether enjoyed as a guilt-free treat or served on special occasions, raw carrot and nut cake demonstrates how wholesome ingredients can be transformed into a delicious dessert that nourishes the body and delights the taste buds.

Chapter 9: Detoxifying Beverages and Herbal Teas Cleansing

Cleansing Wild Berry Juice

Cleansing wild berry juice offers a refreshing and detoxifying beverage that combines the vibrant flavors of assorted berries with cleansing ingredients to support overall health. This juice not only quenches thirst but also provides a range of nutritional benefits from its natural ingredients.

Berries such as strawberries, blueberries, raspberries, and blackberries are rich in antioxidants, vitamins (including vitamin C and vitamin K), and dietary fiber. These nutrients help combat oxidative stress, support immune function, and promote digestive health. Berries also contain natural sugars that provide sweetness without causing a rapid spike in blood sugar levels.

Additional ingredients often found in cleansing wild berry juice include lemon or lime for a citrusy twist and herbs like mint or basil for added flavor and digestive support. Lemon and lime provide vitamin C and citric acid, which aid in detoxification and promote skin health. Fresh herbs contribute antioxidants and anti-inflammatory properties that support overall well-being.

The combination of berries, citrus, and herbs in this juice creates a revitalizing beverage that can be enjoyed as part of a detox regimen or simply as a refreshing drink. Whether served over ice or blended into a smoothie, cleansing wild berry juice offers a delicious way to hydrate the body while supporting its natural detoxification processes.

Herbal Infusion for Digestive Health

An herbal infusion for digestive health is a soothing and therapeutic beverage that combines medicinal herbs known for their digestive benefits. This infusion not only calms the stomach but also promotes overall gastrointestinal wellness through its carefully selected ingredients.

Common herbs used in digestive health infusions include peppermint, chamomile, ginger, and fennel. Peppermint provides relief from indigestion and bloating, while chamomile soothes the stomach and reduces inflammation. Ginger aids in digestion by promoting the production of digestive enzymes and easing nausea. Fennel seeds support digestive motility and help alleviate gas and cramping.

Preparing an herbal infusion involves steeping the selected herbs in hot water to extract their beneficial compounds. This gentle process allows the herbs to release their essential oils and phytonutrients, creating a fragrant and therapeutic beverage that supports digestive comfort and overall well-being.

Herbal infusions for digestive health can be enjoyed hot or cold and are often consumed after meals to aid in digestion. Their natural flavors and soothing properties make them a popular choice for individuals seeking gentle support for digestive issues or simply looking to promote optimal gastrointestinal function.

Sassafras Root Beer

Sassafras root beer offers a unique twist on the classic beverage, utilizing sassafras root bark for its distinctive flavor and potential health benefits. This root beer not only satisfies the palate but also provides a nostalgic taste experience with potential detoxifying properties.

Sassafras, traditionally used by Native American tribes and early European settlers, is known for its aromatic qualities and medicinal properties. The root bark contains essential oils and antioxidants that may support liver health and aid in detoxification processes. However, it's important to note that modern consumption of sassafras is typically without safrole, a compound once present that was found to be carcinogenic in animal studies, leading to its ban in food and beverages.

Modern sassafras root beer recipes often use extracts or flavors derived from sassafras that are safrole-free, ensuring safety for consumption. These recipes combine sassafras flavor with other ingredients such as wintergreen, vanilla, and spices like cinnamon and cloves to create a complex and refreshing beverage.

Sassafras root beer can be enjoyed chilled with ice or as a nostalgic treat on its own. Its unique flavor profile and potential health benefits make it a popular choice for those seeking a twist on traditional soft drinks while exploring historical roots and flavors.

Chapter 10: Probiotic and Prebiotic Recipes from the Past

Homemade Traditional Yogurt

Homemade traditional yogurt is a timeless recipe that has been passed down through generations. It is a rich source of probiotics, which are beneficial bacteria that promote gut health. The process of making yogurt at home is not only cost-effective but also allows for customization in terms of flavor and texture.

To make homemade traditional yogurt, start with high-quality milk. Whole milk is preferred for its creaminess, but you can use low-fat or skim milk if you prefer a lighter version. Begin by heating the milk to about 180°F (82°C). This step is crucial as it kills any unwanted bacteria and helps to denature the proteins in the milk, resulting in a thicker yogurt. Once the milk reaches the desired temperature, let it cool to around 110°F (43°C).

At this point, you will need a starter culture, which can be a few tablespoons of store-bought yogurt with live cultures or a freeze-dried yogurt starter. Add the starter to the cooled milk and mix well. Pour the mixture into jars and incubate it at a steady temperature of about 110°F (43°C) for 4-12 hours. The incubation time will depend on your taste preference; a longer incubation will result in a tangier yogurt. You can use a yogurt maker, an oven with a light on, or a warm spot in your home for incubation.

Once the yogurt has set, refrigerate it for a few hours to firm up further. Homemade yogurt can be enjoyed plain or flavored with fruits, honey, or nuts. It's a versatile ingredient that can be used in smoothies, as a base for dips, or even in baking.

The health benefits of homemade yogurt are numerous. The probiotics it contains help balance the gut microbiome, improving digestion and boosting the immune system. Additionally, yogurt is a good source of calcium, protein, and vitamins B2 and B12. Making yogurt at home also ensures that you avoid additives and preservatives found in many store-bought versions.

Ancient Grains Sourdough Bread

Ancient grains sourdough bread is a wonderful way to incorporate prebiotics into your diet. Prebiotics are non-digestible fibers that feed beneficial bacteria in the gut. Sourdough bread made with ancient grains such as spelt, einkorn, or emmer offers a rich, nutty flavor and a host of nutritional benefits.

To begin, you will need a sourdough starter. This can be made from scratch by mixing flour and water and allowing it to ferment over several days, or you can obtain an established starter from a friend or bakery. Feed the starter with equal parts flour and water daily until it becomes bubbly and active.

For the bread dough, combine the sourdough starter with ancient grain flour, water, and salt. The ratio of flour to water is crucial for the hydration level of the dough, which influences the bread's texture. A higher hydration dough will result in a more open crumb and a chewy texture, while a lower hydration dough will be denser.

Mix the ingredients until they form a rough dough, then let it rest for 30 minutes. This rest period, known as autolyse, allows the flour to fully hydrate and the gluten to develop. After the rest, perform a series of stretch and fold techniques every 30 minutes for a few hours. This process strengthens the gluten network and builds structure in the dough.

Once the dough has developed enough strength, shape it into a round or oval loaf. Place the shaped dough in a proofing basket or bowl lined with a floured cloth and let it ferment at room temperature for several hours, or overnight in the refrigerator for a slower fermentation.

Preheat your oven with a Dutch oven or baking stone inside to 450°F (232°C). When the oven is hot, transfer the dough to the Dutch oven or baking stone, score the top with a sharp knife, and cover with a lid if using a Dutch oven. Bake for 20 minutes with the lid on, then remove the lid and bake for another 20-25 minutes until the crust is deep golden brown and the bread sounds hollow when tapped.

Sourdough bread made with ancient grains is not only delicious but also easier to digest than conventional bread. The long fermentation process breaks down phytic acid, which can inhibit mineral absorption, making the nutrients more bioavailable. The prebiotic fibers in ancient grains support a healthy gut microbiome, contributing to overall digestive health.

Kimchi with Foraged Greens

Kimchi, a traditional Korean fermented vegetable dish, is a powerhouse of probiotics and antioxidants. Incorporating foraged greens into your kimchi adds a unique twist and increases its nutritional value. Foraged greens such as dandelion leaves, nettles, or wild garlic bring diverse flavors and health benefits to this ancient recipe.

To make kimchi with foraged greens, you will need napa cabbage, radishes, garlic, ginger, Korean red pepper flakes (gochugaru), fish sauce or soy sauce, and a selection of foraged greens. Begin by cutting the cabbage into quarters and soaking it in a brine solution of water and salt for several hours. This process draws out excess water from the cabbage and enhances its crispness.

While the cabbage is soaking, prepare the kimchi paste. Blend garlic, ginger, and fish sauce or soy sauce into a smooth paste. Add Korean red pepper flakes to taste; the amount will depend on your desired level of spiciness. Slice the radishes and foraged greens thinly.

After the cabbage has soaked, rinse it thoroughly to remove excess salt and pat it dry. Spread the kimchi paste generously over each cabbage leaf, ensuring even coverage. Mix in the radishes and foraged greens, then pack the mixture tightly into a clean jar or fermentation crock. Leave some space at the top for the kimchi to expand as it ferments.

Cover the jar with a lid or cloth and let it ferment at room temperature for 1-5 days, depending on your preference. Taste the kimchi daily until it reaches your desired level of tanginess. Once it's ready, transfer it to the refrigerator to slow down the fermentation process.

Kimchi with foraged greens offers a unique blend of flavors and an impressive array of health benefits. The fermentation process creates beneficial bacteria that support gut health and boost the immune system. Foraged greens add a variety of vitamins, minerals, and antioxidants, enhancing the nutritional profile of the kimchi. Regular consumption of kimchi can aid digestion, improve heart health, and provide anti-inflammatory benefits.

Incorporating traditional recipes like homemade yogurt, ancient grains sourdough bread, and kimchi with foraged greens into your diet not only supports gut health but also connects you with time-honored culinary practices. These probiotic and prebiotic-rich foods offer a delicious way to nourish your body and promote overall well-being.

Chapter 11: Plant-Based Proteins—A Historical Approach

Lentil and Walnut Loaf

Lentil and walnut loaf is a classic dish that has stood the test of time, celebrated for its rich, earthy flavors and nutritional benefits. This plant-based protein powerhouse has roots in various culinary traditions, showcasing the versatility and nutritional value of lentils and walnuts.

To begin, lentils, particularly green or brown varieties, are the star ingredient. Lentils have been a staple food for centuries, dating back to ancient civilizations in the Near East. They are prized for their high protein content, dietary fiber, and essential nutrients such as iron, folate, and manganese. Walnuts, native to regions surrounding the Mediterranean, add a satisfying crunch and healthy fats, including omega-3 fatty acids, which are crucial for heart health.

To prepare the lentil and walnut loaf, start by cooking the lentils until tender. Simultaneously, finely chop walnuts and toast them in a dry pan to enhance their flavor. The next step involves sautéing a medley of aromatic vegetables such as onions, garlic, carrots, and celery. These vegetables provide a base of savory depth and nutritional value, contributing vitamins A, C, and K, along with various antioxidants.

Combine the cooked lentils, toasted walnuts, and sautéed vegetables in a large mixing bowl. To bind the mixture, add ground flaxseed mixed with water, which acts as a natural egg substitute rich in omega-3 fatty acids and fiber. Season the mixture with herbs like thyme, rosemary, and sage, which have been historically used for their medicinal properties and flavor. Add a splash of tamari or soy sauce for umami depth and a bit of tomato paste for richness.

Transfer the mixture into a loaf pan lined with parchment paper, pressing it down firmly to ensure a cohesive loaf. Bake at 350°F (175°C) for about 45 minutes to an hour, or until the top is golden brown and the loaf is firm to the touch. Allow it to cool slightly before slicing to maintain its structure.

The lentil and walnut loaf is not only a delicious and satisfying meal but also a nutritional powerhouse. Lentils provide a complete protein when combined with grains, essential for muscle repair and growth. Walnuts contribute heart-healthy fats and antioxidants that support brain health and reduce inflammation. This loaf is a testament to the timelessness of plant-based proteins in providing both nourishment and culinary delight.

Nettle and Pea Fritters

Nettle and pea fritters are a historical gem, highlighting the nutritional benefits and culinary versatility of foraged greens and legumes. Nettles, often regarded as a wild superfood, have been used in traditional diets for centuries due to their high vitamin and mineral content. Peas, cultivated since ancient times, are another excellent source of plant-based protein and essential nutrients.

To make nettle and pea fritters, begin by gathering fresh nettles. Nettles are rich in vitamins A, C, and K, as well as minerals such as iron, calcium, and magnesium. Handle them with gloves to avoid their stinging effect, which dissipates once they are cooked. Blanch the nettles in boiling water for a few minutes, then drain and chop them finely.

In a mixing bowl, combine the chopped nettles with cooked peas. Peas provide a sweet, earthy flavor and a good amount of protein and fiber, making them a perfect complement to the nettles. Mash some of the peas to help bind the mixture while leaving some whole for texture.

To add depth of flavor, finely chop onions and garlic and sauté them until golden. Mix these aromatic vegetables into the nettle and pea mixture. For additional binding and a nutritional boost, incorporate chickpea flour, which is high in protein and fiber. Season the mixture with salt, pepper, and a touch of lemon zest for brightness.

Shape the mixture into small patties or fritters. Heat a generous amount of oil in a skillet over medium heat and fry the fritters until golden brown on both sides, about 3-4 minutes per side. The result is a crispy exterior with a tender, flavorful interior.

Nettle and pea fritters are not only delicious but also packed with nutrients. Nettles are known for their anti-inflammatory and antioxidant properties, supporting overall health and well-being. Peas add plant-based protein and fiber, aiding in digestion and maintaining steady blood sugar levels. These fritters celebrate the use of wild and cultivated plant-based ingredients, offering a nutritious and historical perspective on plant-based eating.

Ancient Grain and Vegetable Patties

Ancient grain and vegetable patties are a tribute to the rich culinary traditions that have utilized nutrient-dense grains and vegetables for centuries. Ancient grains such as quinoa, amaranth, and millet are known for their high protein content, fiber, and array of vitamins and minerals. Combined with a variety of vegetables, these patties offer a complete and balanced plant-based meal.

To prepare ancient grain and vegetable patties, start by cooking your choice of ancient grains. Quinoa, amaranth, and millet each bring unique flavors and textures to the patties. Quinoa, for example, is a complete protein, containing all nine essential amino acids, while amaranth is rich in calcium and iron, and millet is a good source of magnesium and phosphorus.

In a large bowl, mix the cooked grains with a selection of finely chopped vegetables. Carrots, bell peppers, zucchini, and spinach are excellent choices, adding color, flavor, and nutrients such as vitamins A, C, and K, as well as folate and fiber. Sauté the vegetables briefly to soften them and enhance their flavors.

To bind the patties, use ground flaxseed mixed with water or chickpea flour, both of which add protein and fiber. Season the mixture with herbs and spices such as cumin, coriander, parsley, and dill, which have been used historically for their medicinal properties and flavor enhancement. A touch of nutritional yeast can also be added for a cheesy, umami flavor and additional B vitamins.

Shape the mixture into patties and cook them in a skillet with a bit of oil over medium heat. Cook until golden brown on each side, about 4-5 minutes per side. Alternatively, the patties can be baked in the oven at 375°F (190°C) for about 20 minutes, flipping halfway through.

Ancient grain and vegetable patties are a versatile and nutritious addition to any meal. They can be served on their own, in a sandwich, or atop a salad. The combination of ancient grains and vegetables provides a well-rounded nutritional profile, offering protein, fiber, vitamins, and minerals essential for maintaining good health.

In conclusion, the historical approach to plant-based proteins through dishes like lentil and walnut loaf, nettle and pea fritters, and ancient grain and vegetable patties showcases the rich culinary traditions and nutritional benefits of plant-based eating. These recipes highlight the timelessness and versatility of plant-based proteins, providing delicious and nutritious meals that have been cherished for generations.

Chapter 12: Anti-Inflammatory Ancient Meals

Turmeric and Ginger Stew

Turmeric and ginger stew is an ancient recipe known for its powerful anti-inflammatory properties. Both turmeric and ginger have been used in traditional medicine for thousands of years, particularly in Ayurvedic and Chinese healing practices. These spices are celebrated not only for their distinct flavors but also for their ability to combat inflammation, which is at the root of many chronic diseases.

To begin making turmeric and ginger stew, gather your ingredients: fresh turmeric root, fresh ginger root, garlic, onions, carrots, sweet potatoes, chickpeas, vegetable broth, coconut milk, and a blend of spices such as cumin, coriander, and black pepper. Turmeric contains curcumin, a compound with potent anti-inflammatory and antioxidant effects, while ginger boasts gingerol, which has similar properties.

Start by finely chopping the onions, garlic, turmeric, and ginger. Sauté them in a large pot with a bit of olive oil until they become fragrant and the onions are translucent. This base of aromatics sets the stage for a richly flavored stew. Add the cumin and coriander, allowing them to toast slightly to release their oils and deepen their flavors.

Next, add the carrots and sweet potatoes, which provide a sweet and earthy counterbalance to the spices. These root vegetables are not only delicious but also packed with vitamins A and C, as well as fiber, which support overall health and immunity. Stir the vegetables to coat them with the spices and aromatics.

Pour in the vegetable broth and coconut milk, bringing the mixture to a simmer. The coconut milk adds a creamy texture and richness to the stew, complementing the spices beautifully. Add the chickpeas, which are an excellent source of plant-based protein and fiber, making the stew hearty and filling.

Allow the stew to simmer for about 30-40 minutes, or until the vegetables are tender. Season with salt and pepper to taste, and don't forget a pinch of black pepper. Black pepper enhances the bioavailability of curcumin, ensuring that your body can absorb and benefit from it more effectively.

Turmeric and ginger stew can be garnished with fresh cilantro and a squeeze of lime juice before serving. The bright, fresh flavors of the garnish cut through the richness of the stew, adding a final touch of vibrancy. This stew is not only delicious and warming but also a powerful ally in reducing inflammation and promoting overall health.

Roasted Chestnuts and Brussels Sprouts

Roasted chestnuts and Brussels sprouts is a dish that brings together the robust, nutty flavors of chestnuts with the slightly bitter, earthy taste of Brussels sprouts. This combination is not only delightful but also offers significant anti-inflammatory benefits. Chestnuts have been consumed since ancient times and were a staple food in many cultures, valued for their high fiber content and rich supply of vitamins and minerals. Brussels sprouts, part of the cruciferous vegetable family, are packed with antioxidants and compounds that support detoxification and reduce inflammation.

To prepare this dish, start by preheating your oven to 400°F (200°C). Gather fresh chestnuts, Brussels sprouts, olive oil, garlic, rosemary, sea salt, and black pepper. Begin by scoring the chestnuts with an 'X' on their flat side. This step is crucial as it prevents them from exploding in the oven and makes them easier to peel once roasted. Spread the chestnuts on a baking sheet and roast them for about 20-25 minutes, or until the shells start to peel back and the chestnuts are tender.

While the chestnuts are roasting, prepare the Brussels sprouts. Trim the ends and remove any yellow or damaged leaves, then cut them in half. In a large bowl, toss the Brussels sprouts with olive oil, minced garlic, fresh rosemary, salt, and pepper. Spread them out on another baking sheet in a single layer.

Once the chestnuts are done, remove them from the oven and let them cool slightly before peeling. The outer shells and the inner brown skin should come off easily, revealing the creamy, sweet chestnut flesh. Add the peeled chestnuts to the baking sheet with the Brussels sprouts and toss to combine.

Return the baking sheet to the oven and roast for another 15-20 minutes, or until the Brussels sprouts are caramelized and tender and the chestnuts have developed a golden-brown exterior. This final roasting step allows the flavors to meld beautifully, creating a dish that is both savory and sweet, with a satisfying crunch from the chestnuts.

Roasted chestnuts and Brussels sprouts are not only a festive and flavorful side dish but also a nutritional powerhouse. Chestnuts are low in fat but high in complex carbohydrates, fiber, and vitamin C, making them a great energy-boosting food. Brussels sprouts are rich in vitamins K and C, folate, and several antioxidants, including kaempferol, which helps reduce inflammation and support overall health. Together, they create a dish that is both delicious and beneficial for reducing inflammation and supporting a healthy diet.

Wild Salmon with Dill and Juniper

Wild salmon with dill and juniper is a dish that harks back to ancient cooking methods, using ingredients that have been prized for their health benefits and culinary qualities for centuries. Wild salmon is an excellent source of omega-3 fatty acids, which are known for their powerful anti-inflammatory properties. Dill and juniper, aromatic herbs used in ancient and traditional cuisines, add unique flavors and additional health benefits.

To prepare wild salmon with dill and juniper, start with fresh, wild-caught salmon fillets. Wild salmon is preferred over farmed salmon for its higher levels of omega-3 fatty acids and lower levels of contaminants. Omega-3 fatty acids are crucial for reducing inflammation in the body, supporting heart and brain health, and maintaining overall cellular function.

Begin by preparing a marinade for the salmon. In a small bowl, mix together fresh dill, crushed juniper berries, lemon juice, olive oil, minced garlic, salt, and pepper. Dill, a herb used since ancient times, is known for its digestive benefits and its ability to soothe the stomach. Juniper berries, used in traditional medicine and cooking, have antimicrobial and anti-inflammatory properties.

Place the salmon fillets in a shallow dish and pour the marinade over them, ensuring they are well-coated. Let the salmon marinate for at least 30 minutes to allow the flavors to penetrate the fish.

Preheat your oven to 375°F (190°C). Line a baking sheet with parchment paper or foil for easy cleanup. Place the marinated salmon fillets on the baking sheet and pour any remaining marinade over the top. Bake the salmon for about 15-20 minutes, or until it is cooked through and flakes easily with a fork.

Serve the wild salmon with a garnish of fresh dill and a few extra juniper berries if desired. The fresh, herbal flavor of the dill complements the rich, buttery taste of the salmon, while the juniper berries add a subtle, piney aroma that enhances the overall dish.

Wild salmon with dill and juniper is not only a delicious and elegant meal but also a nutritional powerhouse. The high levels of omega-3 fatty acids in salmon help reduce inflammation, lower the risk of chronic diseases such as heart disease and arthritis, and support brain health. Dill and juniper add antioxidants and other beneficial compounds that further enhance the anti-inflammatory effects of this dish.

Incorporating ancient meals like turmeric and ginger stew, roasted chestnuts and Brussels sprouts, and wild salmon with dill and juniper into your diet offers a delicious way to harness the power of natural ingredients to reduce inflammation and support overall health. These recipes draw on traditional wisdom and culinary practices, providing not only nutritional benefits but also a connection to the rich history of food as medicine.

Chapter 13: Low-Glycemic Meals from Forgotten Times

Roasted Turnips with Thyme

Roasted turnips with thyme offer a delightful blend of earthy flavors and aromatic herbs, making them a standout dish in low-glycemic cooking. Turnips, known for their crisp texture and slightly peppery taste, are roasted to perfection with fresh thyme, enhancing their natural sweetness without adding unnecessary sugars.

To prepare this dish, start by preheating your oven to 400°F (200°C). Wash and peel the turnips, then cut them into evenly sized cubes or wedges, depending on your preference. Place the turnips on a baking sheet lined with parchment paper or lightly greased with olive oil. Drizzle the turnips with olive oil, ensuring they are coated evenly. Season with salt, freshly ground black pepper, and a generous amount of fresh thyme leaves.

Roast the turnips in the preheated oven for about 25-30 minutes, or until they are tender and golden brown. The high oven temperature helps caramelize the natural sugars in the turnips, enhancing their flavor profile. Once roasted, remove the turnips from the oven and let them cool slightly before serving.

This dish pairs wonderfully with lean proteins such as grilled chicken or fish, providing a balanced meal that is rich in flavor and low on the glycemic index. The combination of roasted turnips and thyme not only satisfies your taste buds but also supports your nutritional goals by offering a satisfying alternative to higher glycemic side dishes.

Venison and Barberry Stew

Venison and barberry stew is a hearty and nourishing dish that harkens back to traditional cooking methods, focusing on wholesome ingredients with low glycemic impact. Venison, a lean and protein-rich meat, is simmered to tenderness alongside tart barberries, creating a unique flavor profile that is both savory and slightly tangy.

To prepare this stew, start by browning the venison in a large pot with a small amount of olive oil over medium-high heat. Browning the meat adds depth of flavor to the stew. Once browned, remove the venison from the pot and set it aside.

In the same pot, add diced onions, carrots, and celery, sautéing them until they are softened and aromatic. Return the venison to the pot and add low-sodium beef broth, enough to cover the meat and vegetables. Bring the stew to a boil, then reduce the heat to low and let it simmer gently for about 1.5 to 2 hours, or until the venison is tender.

About 30 minutes before serving, add dried barberries to the stew. Barberries are small, tart berries that add a distinctive flavor and vibrant color to the dish. Simmer the stew uncovered until the barberries are plump and tender. Season with salt, pepper, and a pinch of ground cinnamon or allspice for added warmth.

Serve the venison and barberry stew hot, garnished with fresh parsley or thyme for a burst of freshness. This dish is not only low on the glycemic index but also high in protein, making it a satisfying choice for those looking to maintain stable blood sugar levels while enjoying a comforting meal.

Pearled Barley Risotto with Wild Mushrooms

Pearled barley risotto with wild mushrooms is a nutritious and flavorful alternative to traditional rice-based risotto, offering a low-glycemic option that is rich in fiber and complex carbohydrates. Barley, known for its chewy texture and nutty flavor, absorbs the savory essence of wild mushrooms, creating a creamy and indulgent dish without the high glycemic load.

To prepare this risotto, begin by rinsing pearled barley under cold water to remove any excess starch. In a large saucepan, heat a tablespoon of olive oil over medium heat. Add finely chopped shallots or garlic, sautéing them until they become translucent and fragrant.

Add the pearled barley to the saucepan, stirring constantly to coat the grains with the oil and aromatics. This helps to toast the barley slightly, enhancing its nutty flavor. Deglaze the pan with a splash of dry white wine, allowing it to simmer until most of the liquid has evaporated.

Gradually add low-sodium vegetable or chicken broth to the barley, one ladleful at a time, stirring frequently and allowing each addition to be absorbed before adding more. This slow-cooking process helps release the barley's starches, creating a creamy texture reminiscent of traditional risotto.

Meanwhile, in a separate skillet, sauté a variety of wild mushrooms such as shiitake, oyster, or porcini in a bit of olive oil until they are tender and golden brown. Season with salt, pepper, and a pinch of fresh thyme or rosemary for added depth of flavor.

Once the barley is tender and creamy, stir in the sautéed mushrooms and a generous handful of grated Parmesan cheese. The cheese adds richness and umami to the dish, complementing the earthy flavors of the mushrooms and barley.

Serve the pearled barley risotto with wild mushrooms immediately, garnished with chopped parsley or chives for a burst of freshness. This dish is a wonderful example of low-glycemic cooking that doesn't compromise on taste or satisfaction, making it suitable for those seeking balanced meals that support stable blood sugar levels.

These recipes from "Low-Glycemic Meals from Forgotten Times" highlight the versatility of ingredients and culinary techniques that prioritize low-glycemic index foods without sacrificing flavor or nutritional value. Each dish offers a unique combination of flavors and textures, showcasing how traditional cooking methods can be adapted to meet modern dietary preferences and health goals.

Chapter 14: Heart-Healthy Historical Recipes

Foraged Berry Compote

Foraged berry compote is a delightful and heart-healthy dessert that celebrates the natural sweetness of berries while providing essential nutrients and antioxidants beneficial for cardiovascular health. This recipe draws inspiration from traditional methods of preserving fruits, ensuring that the berries retain their flavors and nutritional benefits without added sugars.

To prepare this compote, start by gathering a variety of fresh berries such as strawberries, blueberries, raspberries, and blackberries. If available, include wild berries for their unique flavors and higher antioxidant content. Rinse the berries thoroughly under cold water and pat them dry with a clean towel.

In a saucepan, combine the berries with a splash of water or freshly squeezed orange juice to enhance their natural sweetness. Bring the mixture to a gentle simmer over medium heat, stirring occasionally to prevent sticking. As the berries heat up, they will release their juices, creating a fragrant and flavorful compote.

To add complexity to the compote, consider incorporating aromatic spices such as cinnamon sticks or a dash of freshly grated nutmeg. These spices not only complement the berries but also provide additional antioxidant benefits and heart-healthy properties.

Simmer the berry mixture for about 10-15 minutes, or until the berries have softened and the liquid has thickened to a syrupy consistency. Taste the compote and adjust the sweetness by adding a drizzle of honey or maple syrup if desired, although the natural sweetness of the berries often suffices.

Once the compote has cooled slightly, transfer it to a serving bowl or individual dessert dishes. Serve the foraged berry compote warm or chilled, garnished with a sprig of fresh mint or a dollop of Greek yogurt for added creaminess and protein. This versatile dessert can also be enjoyed as a topping for oatmeal, yogurt parfaits, or whole-grain pancakes, making it a nutritious addition to any heart-healthy meal plan.

Grilled Trout with Wild Herbs

Grilled trout with wild herbs is a nutritious and heart-healthy dish that showcases the delicate flavor of fresh fish enhanced by aromatic herbs and a hint of smokiness from the grill. Trout, rich in omega-3 fatty acids and lean protein, is grilled to perfection alongside a medley of wild herbs, offering a satisfying meal that supports cardiovascular health.

To prepare this dish, start by cleaning and gutting fresh trout, ensuring that it is scaled and thoroughly rinsed under cold water. Pat the trout dry with paper towels and lightly brush both sides with olive oil to prevent sticking during grilling. Season generously with salt and freshly ground black pepper.

Preheat your grill to medium-high heat and lightly oil the grates to prevent the fish from sticking. Place the trout on the grill, skin side down, and cook for approximately 4-5 minutes per side, or until the flesh flakes easily with a fork. Avoid overcooking the trout to retain its moisture and delicate texture.

While the trout is grilling, prepare the wild herb mixture. Combine chopped fresh herbs such as parsley, dill, chives, and thyme in a small bowl. Add a drizzle of olive oil, a squeeze of fresh lemon juice, and a pinch of salt to the herbs, tossing gently to combine. This herb mixture adds brightness and herbal notes to complement the grilled trout.

Once the trout is cooked through, transfer it to a serving platter and generously sprinkle the grilled fish with the wild herb mixture. The heat from the trout will slightly wilt the herbs, releasing their aromas and flavors. Serve the grilled trout with a wedge of lemon for an extra burst of citrusy freshness.

This heart-healthy dish is low in saturated fats and high in omega-3 fatty acids, making it an excellent choice for maintaining cardiovascular health. Pair the grilled trout with a side of steamed vegetables or a whole-grain salad for a well-rounded meal that is as nutritious as it is delicious.

Roasted Nuts with Sea Salt and Olive Oil

Roasted nuts with sea salt and olive oil are a satisfying and heart-healthy snack that combines the natural crunch of nuts with the savory richness of olive oil and a hint of sea salt. This recipe highlights the nutritional benefits of nuts, which are packed with healthy fats, protein, and essential nutrients that support heart health.

To prepare this snack, start by selecting a variety of raw nuts such as almonds, walnuts, pecans, and cashews. Spread the nuts evenly on a baking sheet lined with parchment paper, ensuring they are in a single layer for even roasting. Drizzle the nuts with extra-virgin olive oil, using your hands to toss them until they are evenly coated.

Sprinkle the nuts with a pinch of sea salt, adjusting the amount to your preference. Sea salt not only enhances the flavors of the nuts but also provides trace minerals that are beneficial for overall health. You can also add a sprinkle of dried herbs such as rosemary or thyme for an extra layer of flavor.

Roast the nuts in a preheated oven at 350°F (175°C) for about 10-15 minutes, stirring halfway through to ensure even cooking. Keep a close eye on the nuts to prevent them from burning, as they can quickly go from perfectly roasted to overdone.

Once the nuts are golden brown and fragrant, remove them from the oven and let them cool completely on the baking sheet. As they cool, the nuts will become crispier, making them perfect for snacking. Transfer the roasted nuts to an airtight container or Mason jar for storage.

Enjoy the roasted nuts with sea salt and olive oil as a standalone snack or incorporate them into salads, yogurt parfaits, or trail mixes for added crunch and nutrition. This heart-healthy snack is ideal for satisfying cravings while providing essential nutrients that support cardiovascular health.

These recipes from "Heart-Healthy Historical Recipes" showcase the diversity of ingredients and cooking techniques that prioritize heart health without compromising on flavor or satisfaction. Each dish offers a unique combination of wholesome ingredients and culinary traditions, making them suitable choices for anyone looking to maintain a heart-healthy diet.

Chapter 15: Gluten-Free Eating from Antiquity

Buckwheat Crepes with Honeyed Fruit

Buckwheat crepes with honeyed fruit are a delightful gluten-free twist on a classic dish, showcasing the nutty flavor of buckwheat flour paired with naturally sweetened fruits. Buckwheat, despite its name, is not related to wheat and is naturally gluten-free, making it an excellent choice for those with gluten sensitivities.

To prepare buckwheat crepes, start by combining buckwheat flour, eggs, milk (or a dairy-free alternative), and a pinch of salt in a mixing bowl. Whisk the ingredients together until you achieve a smooth batter. Let the batter rest for about 15-20 minutes to allow the flour to hydrate.

While the batter is resting, prepare the honeyed fruit topping. Choose a variety of fresh fruits such as strawberries, blueberries, raspberries, and thinly sliced apples or pears. In a small saucepan, gently heat honey or maple syrup until it becomes liquid. Toss the fruits in the warm honey or syrup until they are coated evenly.

Heat a non-stick skillet or crepe pan over medium heat and lightly grease it with butter or coconut oil. Pour a ladleful of the buckwheat batter into the center of the skillet, swirling it gently to spread the batter thinly and evenly. Cook the crepe for about 1-2 minutes on each side, or until it is golden brown and cooked through.

Repeat the process with the remaining batter, stacking the cooked crepes on a plate and covering them with a clean kitchen towel to keep them warm. Once all the crepes are cooked, spoon the honeyed fruit mixture onto each crepe, folding or rolling them as desired.

Serve the buckwheat crepes with honeyed fruit warm, drizzled with any remaining honey or syrup from the fruit mixture. This dish makes for a delicious breakfast or dessert option that is not only gluten-free but also packed with fiber, vitamins, and antioxidants from the fresh fruits.

Amaranth Pilaf with Roasted Squash

Amaranth pilaf with roasted squash is a hearty and nutritious dish that highlights the ancient grain amaranth, known for its high protein content and gluten-free properties. Amaranth has a slightly nutty flavor and a chewy texture, making it a versatile ingredient in both savory and sweet dishes.

To prepare amaranth pilaf, start by rinsing the amaranth under cold water to remove any bitterness. In a saucepan, combine the rinsed amaranth with double the amount of water or broth (e.g., 1 cup of amaranth to 2 cups of water). Bring the mixture to a boil over medium-high heat, then reduce the heat to low and cover the saucepan with a lid.

Simmer the amaranth for about 20-25 minutes, or until all the liquid is absorbed and the grains are tender. Fluff the cooked amaranth with a fork to separate the grains and let it cool slightly.

Meanwhile, prepare the roasted squash. Choose a variety of winter squash such as butternut or acorn squash, peeling and cubing them into bite-sized pieces. Toss the squash cubes with olive oil, salt, and a sprinkle of your favorite herbs or spices such as rosemary or paprika.

Roast the squash in a preheated oven at 400°F (200°C) for about 20-25 minutes, or until the squash is tender and caramelized around the edges. Remove the roasted squash from the oven and let it cool slightly.

Combine the cooked amaranth with the roasted squash in a large serving bowl, gently folding them together to mix. Adjust the seasoning with salt and pepper to taste, adding a drizzle of extra-virgin olive oil for richness.

Serve the amaranth pilaf with roasted squash warm as a main dish or hearty side, garnished with fresh herbs such as parsley or cilantro for added freshness. This gluten-free recipe is not only satisfying but also packed with nutrients that support overall health and well-being.

Chestnut Flour Brownies

Chestnut flour brownies are a decadent gluten-free dessert that combines the rich flavor of chestnut flour with dark chocolate, creating a fudgy and indulgent treat. Chestnut flour, made from ground dried chestnuts, adds a sweet and nutty flavor to baked goods while remaining gluten-free and nutrient-dense.

To prepare chestnut flour brownies, start by preheating your oven to 350°F (175°C) and lining a baking dish with parchment paper or greasing it lightly with coconut oil.

In a mixing bowl, combine chestnut flour, cocoa powder, baking soda, and a pinch of salt. Whisk the dry ingredients together until they are well combined and free of lumps.

In a separate bowl, melt dark chocolate and unsalted butter together over low heat or in the microwave, stirring frequently until smooth and combined. Allow the chocolate mixture to cool slightly before proceeding.

Add eggs, vanilla extract, and honey or maple syrup to the melted chocolate mixture, stirring until smooth and creamy. Gradually add the dry ingredients to the wet ingredients, mixing until just combined. Be careful not to overmix the batter, as this can result in dense brownies.

Fold in chopped nuts such as walnuts or pecans if desired, adding a crunchy texture and additional nutrients to the brownies.

Pour the brownie batter into the prepared baking dish, spreading it evenly with a spatula. Bake the brownies in the preheated oven for 20-25 minutes, or until the edges are set and a toothpick inserted into the center comes out with a few moist crumbs.

Remove the brownies from the oven and let them cool completely in the baking dish before slicing them into squares. Dust the cooled brownies with cocoa powder or powdered sugar for a decorative touch.

Enjoy the chestnut flour brownies as a decadent gluten-free dessert, perfect for satisfying chocolate cravings while providing the nutritional benefits of chestnut flour. These brownies are sure to be a hit with gluten-free and non-gluten-free eaters alike, showcasing the versatility and deliciousness of alternative flours in baking.

These recipes from "Gluten-Free Eating from Antiquity" demonstrate the richness and versatility of gluten-free ingredients such as buckwheat, amaranth, and chestnut flour. Each dish offers a flavorful and nutritious option that celebrates ancient grains while catering to modern dietary preferences and health needs.

Chapter 16: Brain Foods from the Lost Pages

Brain Foods from the Lost Pages

In this chapter, we delve into the exquisite realm of brain-nourishing foods that have been revered through ages for their cognitive benefits. These culinary treasures not only tantalize the taste buds but also provide a bounty of nutrients that support mental clarity, focus, and overall brain health. Let's explore the recipes and their nutritional benefits:

Walnut and Pomegranate Salad

The Walnut and Pomegranate Salad is a vibrant blend of flavors and textures that harmoniously come together to create a dish as visually appealing as it is nutritious. Walnuts, known for their brain-boosting omega-3 fatty acids, provide essential nutrients like alpha-linolenic acid (ALA) and antioxidants that support cognitive function. Pomegranate seeds, prized for their antioxidant prowess, add a burst of tangy sweetness along with beneficial polyphenols that promote brain health by protecting against oxidative stress. The salad's fresh greens, such as spinach or arugula, contribute folate, vitamin K, and other micronutrients crucial for brain function and overall well-being.

Grilled Mackerel with Lemon Balm

Grilled Mackerel with Lemon Balm combines the richness of omega-3 fatty acids from mackerel with the subtle citrusy aroma of lemon balm, a herb historically valued for its calming effects on the mind. Mackerel's omega-3s, particularly docosahexaenoic acid (DHA), are essential for brain health, playing a crucial role in neuronal structure and function. Lemon balm, renowned for its potential to reduce anxiety and improve mood, adds a refreshing twist to the dish while potentially supporting cognitive performance through its antioxidant properties. This dish not only satisfies the palate but also nourishes the brain with every savory bite.

Beetroot and Blueberry Mash

The Beetroot and Blueberry Mash is a delightful symphony of colors and flavors, marrying the earthy sweetness of beetroots with the tangy burst of blueberries. Beetroots, rich in nitrates that enhance blood flow to the brain, may improve cognitive function by promoting cerebral circulation. Their vibrant hue signifies a high content of betalains, potent antioxidants that protect brain cells from oxidative damage. Blueberries, dubbed as "brain berries," are packed with flavonoids like anthocyanins that have been linked to improved memory and cognitive function. Together, these ingredients create a mash that not only nourishes the brain but also delights the senses with its robust flavors and nutritional benefits.

Each of these recipes not only offers a culinary journey but also provides a gateway to enhancing cognitive health through the power of nutrient-dense foods. Incorporating these dishes into your diet can contribute to long-term brain health and vitality, making them essential additions to any wellness-focused menu.

Chapter 17: Beauty Recipes from Historical Traditions

Beauty Recipes from Historical Traditions

Discover the timeless allure of ancient beauty rituals with recipes that have transcended generations, celebrated for their rejuvenating properties and natural efficacy. From facial masks to soothing bath soaks, these historical treasures offer a holistic approach to skincare that combines luxurious ingredients with age-old wisdom. Let's explore the recipes and their beauty-enhancing benefits:

Cucumber and Mint Facial Mask (Edible and Topical)

The Cucumber and Mint Facial Mask embodies the refreshing essence of nature's bounty, combining cooling cucumber with invigorating mint for a dual-purpose treat for both internal and external beauty. Cucumbers, renowned for their hydrating and soothing properties, are rich in vitamins C and K, silica, and antioxidants that nourish and rejuvenate the skin. Mint, prized for its aromatic freshness and skin-cleansing properties, adds a revitalizing touch while potentially soothing irritation and promoting a clearer complexion. This mask can be applied topically to refresh and tone the skin or enjoyed internally for a dual beauty boost that radiates from within.

Pomegranate and Honey Scrub

The Pomegranate and Honey Scrub offers a luxurious blend of exfoliation and hydration, harnessing the antioxidant-rich power of pomegranate seeds and the moisturizing properties of honey. Pomegranates, revered for their potent antioxidant content, including punicalagins and anthocyanins, help protect the skin from environmental damage while promoting a youthful glow. Honey, a natural humectant, locks in moisture and gently exfoliates the skin, revealing a smoother texture and enhancing overall radiance. Together, these ingredients create a scrub that not only buffs away dead skin cells but also nourishes and revitalizes, leaving the skin supple and luminous.

Oatmeal and Lavender Bath Soak

The Oatmeal and Lavender Bath Soak invites you to indulge in a sensory retreat that calms the mind and rejuvenates the body, drawing inspiration from ancient practices of relaxation and rejuvenation. Oatmeal, celebrated for its soothing properties and ability to relieve dryness and irritation, forms the base of this nourishing bath soak. Lavender, prized for its calming aroma and skin-soothing benefits, promotes relaxation while potentially reducing inflammation and promoting skin healing. This bath soak not only provides hydration and relief for dry or sensitive skin but also creates a tranquil spa-like experience that enhances overall well-being.

These beauty recipes from historical traditions offer more than just skincare; they embody a connection to nature and a commitment to nurturing beauty through time-honored ingredients and practices. Incorporating these rituals into your skincare regimen allows you to experience the luxurious benefits of natural beauty treatments while honoring centuries of wisdom and tradition.

Chapter 18: Family Meals from Lost Cultures

Embark on a culinary journey through lost cultures with recipes that evoke the warmth of family gatherings and the rich tapestry of diverse culinary traditions. These hearty meals not only nourish the body but also celebrate the heritage and flavors of ancient civilizations. Let's delve into the recipes and their cultural significance:

Roast Duck with Apples and Root Vegetables

Roast Duck with Apples and Root Vegetables is a dish that pays homage to traditions of roasting meats and incorporating seasonal fruits and vegetables in culinary practices. Duck, prized for its rich flavor and tender meat, is complemented by the sweetness of apples and the earthy richness of root vegetables such as carrots, parsnips, and potatoes. This combination not only creates a balanced and satisfying meal but also reflects the ingenuity of ancient cooks who utilized local ingredients to create nourishing family feasts. The dish is often seasoned with herbs and spices that enhance the flavors, making it a centerpiece that brings generations together around the dinner table.

Baked Millet and Vegetables in Clay Pots

Baked Millet and Vegetables in Clay Pots offers a glimpse into ancient cooking methods and the nutritional wisdom of incorporating whole grains and seasonal vegetables into everyday meals. Millet, a staple in many ancient cultures due to its versatility and nutrient density, forms the heart of this dish, providing a hearty base that's both filling and nutritious. Seasonal vegetables such as tomatoes, bell peppers, and zucchini add color, flavor, and a variety of vitamins and minerals essential for well-rounded nutrition. Baking the dish in clay pots not only imparts a unique flavor but also harkens back to traditional cooking practices that emphasize slow, even cooking for maximum flavor and nutrient retention. This wholesome meal not only satisfies hunger but also connects families to their culinary heritage through time-honored ingredients and cooking techniques.

Steamed Fish with Fermented Black Beans

Steamed Fish with Fermented Black Beans showcases the art of steaming, a cooking method revered for preserving the delicate flavors and textures of seafood while infusing it with aromatic seasonings. Fish, cherished for its lean protein and omega-3 fatty acids essential for heart health, is delicately steamed to perfection, ensuring tender, moist flesh that melts in the mouth. Fermented black beans, a staple in Asian cuisines, add depth and umami to the dish, while ingredients like ginger, garlic, and soy sauce contribute layers of flavor that complement the natural sweetness of the fish. This dish not only exemplifies the culinary finesse of ancient cultures but also honors the simplicity and elegance of steamed preparations that have stood the test of time.

These family meals from lost cultures invite you to savor the flavors and stories of ancient civilizations through dishes that nourish both body and soul. By embracing these recipes, you not only celebrate culinary diversity but also preserve the culinary legacies passed down through generations.

Chapter 19: Herbal Teas and Decoctions

Wild Rosehip and Hibiscus Tea

Wild Rosehip and Hibiscus Tea is a vibrant, tangy blend that not only delights the senses but also provides numerous health benefits. Rosehips, the fruit of the wild rose plant, are packed with vitamin C, antioxidants, and anti-inflammatory compounds, making them a powerful ally for boosting the immune system, promoting skin health, and reducing inflammation. Hibiscus flowers, known for their deep red color, are rich in antioxidants, particularly flavonoids, and have been shown to lower blood pressure, improve liver health, and aid in weight loss. Combining these two ingredients creates a tea that is not only delicious but also highly beneficial for overall health.

To prepare Wild Rosehip and Hibiscus Tea, start by sourcing high-quality dried rosehips and hibiscus flowers. You can find these at health food stores, specialty tea shops, or online. Ensure that the ingredients are organic and free from additives or preservatives. For a single serving, you will need about one tablespoon of dried rosehips and one tablespoon of dried hibiscus flowers.

Begin by boiling water in a kettle or pot. While the water is heating, place the dried rosehips and hibiscus flowers into a teapot or a heatproof container. Once the water reaches a rolling boil, pour it over the dried ingredients. Cover the teapot or container with a lid or a small plate to trap the steam and allow the herbs to steep. Steep the tea for at least 10-15 minutes to ensure that the beneficial compounds are fully extracted. For a stronger flavor, you can steep it for up to 30 minutes.

After steeping, strain the tea to remove the solid pieces. The resulting liquid should be a beautiful deep red color with a tart, fruity aroma. You can enjoy the tea hot or let it cool down and serve it over ice for a refreshing iced tea. If you prefer a sweeter taste, consider adding a natural sweetener like honey, agave syrup, or stevia. However, be mindful of the added calories and potential blood sugar spikes if you are managing your weight or blood sugar levels.

Drinking Wild Rosehip and Hibiscus Tea regularly can provide numerous health benefits. The high vitamin C content in rosehips can boost your immune system, helping your body fight off infections and illnesses. Vitamin C is also essential for collagen production, which is crucial for maintaining healthy skin, joints, and blood vessels. The antioxidants in both rosehips and hibiscus help neutralize free radicals, reducing oxidative stress and lowering the risk of chronic diseases such as heart disease, diabetes, and cancer.

Hibiscus has been studied for its ability to lower blood pressure. Several studies have shown that drinking hibiscus tea can significantly reduce both systolic and diastolic blood pressure in people with hypertension. This effect is attributed to the tea's ability to relax blood vessels and improve blood flow. Additionally, hibiscus has been found to have diuretic properties, which can help reduce fluid retention and further lower blood pressure.

The anti-inflammatory properties of rosehips can help reduce inflammation in the body, which is linked to numerous chronic diseases. Regular consumption of rosehip tea has been shown to reduce markers of inflammation, such as C-reactive protein (CRP), and improve symptoms of osteoarthritis, such as joint pain and stiffness.

Hibiscus tea has also been studied for its potential to improve liver health. The antioxidants in hibiscus can help protect the liver from damage caused by free radicals and toxins. Some studies have shown that hibiscus extract can reduce liver damage and improve liver function in people with fatty liver disease.

In addition to its health benefits, Wild Rosehip and Hibiscus Tea is a versatile beverage that can be enjoyed in various ways. You can use it as a base for herbal blends by adding other herbs and spices such as mint, ginger, or cinnamon. You can also use it as a base for fruit punches or cocktails, adding a unique flavor and health benefits to your drinks.

In summary, Wild Rosehip and Hibiscus Tea is a delicious and healthful beverage that offers numerous benefits. By incorporating this tea into your daily routine, you can boost your immune system, improve your skin health, lower your blood pressure, and reduce inflammation. Its vibrant color and tangy flavor make it a delightful drink that can be enjoyed hot or cold, and it can be easily customized to suit your taste preferences.

Dandelion and Burdock Root Brew

Dandelion and Burdock Root Brew is a traditional herbal tea known for its detoxifying and liver-supporting properties. Dandelion root is rich in vitamins and minerals, including vitamins A, C, and K, as well as iron, calcium, and potassium. It has been used for centuries to support liver health, improve digestion, and promote detoxification. Burdock root, another powerful detoxifying herb, is known for its ability to purify the blood, support kidney function, and improve skin health. Together, these two roots create a potent brew that can help cleanse the body, support liver function, and promote overall health and well-being.

To prepare Dandelion and Burdock Root Brew, you will need dried dandelion root and dried burdock root. These can be found at health food stores, herbal shops, or online. Ensure that the roots are organic and free from additives or preservatives. For a single serving, you will need about one tablespoon of dried dandelion root and one tablespoon of dried burdock root.

Start by bringing a pot of water to a boil. While the water is heating, place the dried roots into a teapot or a heatproof container. Once the water reaches a rolling boil, pour it over the dried roots. Cover the teapot or container with a lid or a small plate to trap the steam and allow the herbs to steep. Steep the brew for at least 15-20 minutes to ensure that the beneficial compounds are fully extracted. For a stronger flavor and more potent effects, you can steep it for up to 45 minutes.

After steeping, strain the brew to remove the solid pieces. The resulting liquid should have a rich, earthy flavor with a slightly bitter taste. You can enjoy the brew hot or let it cool down and serve it over ice. If you prefer a sweeter taste, consider adding a natural sweetener like honey, agave syrup, or stevia. You can also add a splash of lemon juice to enhance the flavor and boost the detoxifying effects.

Drinking Dandelion and Burdock Root Brew regularly can provide numerous health benefits. Dandelion root is known for its ability to support liver health. It stimulates bile production, which helps the liver process and eliminate toxins from the body. This can improve digestion, reduce bloating, and promote healthy liver function. Dandelion root also has diuretic properties, which can help reduce fluid retention and support kidney function.

Burdock root is a powerful blood purifier. It helps remove toxins from the bloodstream, which can improve skin health and reduce the risk of chronic diseases. Burdock root is also known for its anti-inflammatory properties, which can help reduce inflammation in the body and alleviate symptoms of conditions such as arthritis and eczema.

The combination of dandelion and burdock roots makes this brew a potent detoxifier. Regular consumption can help cleanse the body of toxins, support liver and kidney function, and promote overall health and well-being. It can also help improve digestion, reduce bloating, and support healthy skin.

In addition to its detoxifying properties, Dandelion and Burdock Root Brew is a versatile beverage that can be enjoyed in various ways. You can use it as a base for herbal blends by adding other herbs and spices such as ginger, cinnamon, or licorice root. You can also use it as a base for soups or stews, adding a unique flavor and health benefits to your meals.

In summary, Dandelion and Burdock Root Brew is a powerful herbal tea that offers numerous health benefits. By incorporating this brew into your daily routine, you can support liver health, improve digestion, detoxify your body, and promote overall health and well-being. Its rich, earthy flavor and detoxifying properties make it a valuable addition to any wellness regimen.

Pine Needle and Citrus Tea for Immunity

Pine Needle and Citrus Tea is a refreshing and immune-boosting beverage that combines the benefits of pine needles and citrus fruits. Pine needles are rich in vitamin C, antioxidants, and other compounds that support immune function, improve respiratory health, and promote overall well-being. Citrus fruits, such as lemons, oranges, and grapefruits, are also high in vitamin C and other antioxidants that help strengthen the immune system, reduce inflammation, and protect against infections. Together, these ingredients create a powerful tea that can help boost immunity, improve respiratory health, and enhance overall vitality.

To prepare Pine Needle and Citrus Tea, you will need fresh pine needles and fresh citrus fruits. Pine needles can be sourced from certain species of pine trees, such as Eastern White Pine or Ponderosa Pine. Ensure that the pine needles are free from pesticides and other contaminants. For the citrus fruits, you can use a combination of lemons, oranges, and grapefruits, depending on your taste preferences. For a single serving, you will need about one tablespoon of chopped pine needles and the juice of one lemon or half an orange or grapefruit.

Begin by washing the pine needles thoroughly to remove any dirt or debris. Chop the pine needles into small pieces to help release their beneficial compounds. Next, bring a pot of water to a boil. While the water is heating, place the chopped pine needles into a teapot or a heatproof container. Once the water reaches a rolling boil, pour it over the pine needles. Cover the teapot or container with a lid or a small plate to trap the steam and allow the needles to steep. Steep the tea for at least 10-15 minutes to ensure that the beneficial compounds are fully extracted.

While the pine needles are steeping, juice the citrus

fruits to extract their juice. You can use a citrus juicer or simply squeeze the fruits by hand. Once the pine needle tea has finished steeping, strain it to remove the solid pieces. Add the freshly squeezed citrus juice to the strained tea and stir well. The resulting tea should have a bright, citrusy flavor with a hint of pine.

You can enjoy Pine Needle and Citrus Tea hot or let it cool down and serve it over ice for a refreshing iced tea. If you prefer a sweeter taste, you can add a natural sweetener like honey or agave syrup. Avoid adding sugar or artificial sweeteners, as they can negate some of the health benefits of the tea.

Drinking Pine Needle and Citrus Tea regularly can provide numerous health benefits. The high vitamin C content in both pine needles and citrus fruits helps boost the immune system, making it easier for your body to fight off infections and illnesses. Vitamin C is also essential for collagen production, which is important for maintaining healthy skin, joints, and blood vessels.

Pine needles have been traditionally used to support respiratory health. They have expectorant properties, which can help loosen mucus and phlegm from the respiratory tract, making it easier to breathe. Pine needle tea is often used as a natural remedy for coughs, colds, and respiratory infections. The antioxidants in pine needles also help reduce inflammation and oxidative stress in the body, which can contribute to overall health and well-being.

Citrus fruits are known for their antioxidant properties, which help protect cells from damage caused by free radicals. This can reduce inflammation, lower the risk of chronic diseases, and promote overall longevity. Citrus fruits also contain flavonoids, which have anti-inflammatory and immune-boosting effects.

In addition to its health benefits, Pine Needle and Citrus Tea is a flavorful and versatile beverage. You can experiment with different combinations of citrus fruits and pine needles to create unique variations of the tea. You can also add other herbs and spices such as ginger or cinnamon to enhance the flavor and health benefits.

In summary, Pine Needle and Citrus Tea is a refreshing and immune-boosting beverage that offers numerous health benefits. By incorporating this tea into your daily routine, you can boost your immune system, improve respiratory health, and enhance overall vitality. Its bright, citrusy flavor and medicinal properties make it a valuable addition to any wellness regimen.

Chapter 20: Seasonal Recipes

Spring Foraged Salad with Violets and Sorrel

Spring Foraged Salad with Violets and Sorrel celebrates the bounty of early spring with fresh, wild ingredients that awaken the palate and nourish the body. Violets, known for their delicate purple flowers, are not just a beautiful addition to the plate but also rich in vitamins A and C, antioxidants, and anti-inflammatory compounds. Sorrel, with its lemony tang, adds brightness and a burst of flavor, along with vitamins B6 and C, potassium, and magnesium. Combined with other foraged greens and edible flowers, this salad is a celebration of the season's new growth and vitality.

To prepare Spring Foraged Salad with Violets and Sorrel, start by gathering fresh violets and sorrel from a clean, pesticide-free area. Ensure that the flowers and leaves are free from dirt and insects by gently rinsing them under cold water and patting them dry with a clean towel. You can also add other spring greens such as dandelion greens, chickweed, or young nettle leaves for variety and added nutrition.

For the dressing, whisk together extra virgin olive oil, freshly squeezed lemon juice, a touch of honey or maple syrup for sweetness, and a pinch of sea salt and freshly ground black pepper to taste. This simple dressing enhances the flavors of the delicate greens without overpowering them.

Once your ingredients are prepared, gently toss the violets, sorrel, and other spring greens in a large salad bowl. Drizzle the dressing over the salad and toss again until evenly coated. Garnish with additional violets or edible flowers for an elegant touch.

Spring Foraged Salad with Violets and Sorrel not only delights the senses but also provides a wealth of health benefits. Violets are rich in antioxidants that help combat oxidative stress and inflammation in the body. They also contain vitamins A and C, which support immune function and skin health. Sorrel's lemony flavor adds a refreshing twist to the salad while providing vitamins B6 and C, potassium, and magnesium, which are essential for overall health and vitality.

This salad is a perfect way to celebrate the arrival of spring and the abundance of fresh, wild ingredients that nature provides. It can be served as a light lunch or a side dish alongside grilled chicken or fish. Its vibrant colors and flavors will impress your guests and nourish your body with seasonal goodness.

Summer Fruit Tart with Ancient Grain Crust

Summer Fruit Tart with Ancient Grain Crust is a delightful dessert that showcases the sweetness and abundance of summer fruits while offering a wholesome, nutrient-dense crust made from ancient grains. Ancient grains such as spelt, einkorn, or kamut are known for their rich nutritional profiles, including higher protein content and a broader range of vitamins and minerals compared to modern wheat. This tart combines the natural sweetness of ripe summer fruits with the nutty flavor and wholesome goodness of an ancient grain crust, creating a dessert that is both indulgent and nourishing.

To prepare the Ancient Grain Crust, start by combining ancient grain flour (such as spelt or einkorn flour), almond flour, a pinch of sea salt, and a tablespoon of coconut sugar in a mixing bowl. Cut cold unsalted butter or coconut oil into the flour mixture until it resembles coarse crumbs. Add cold water, a tablespoon at a time, and mix until the dough comes together. Press the dough evenly into a tart pan or pie dish, making sure to cover the bottom and sides. Prick the bottom of the crust with a fork to prevent air bubbles from forming during baking.

Pre-bake the crust in a preheated oven at 350°F (175°C) for about 15-20 minutes or until lightly golden brown. Let it cool completely before filling.

For the filling, choose a variety of ripe summer fruits such as berries, peaches, apricots, or figs. Arrange the fruits attractively over the cooled crust. You can brush the fruits with a light glaze made from warmed apricot jam or honey for added shine and sweetness.

Serve the Summer Fruit Tart with Ancient Grain Crust chilled or at room temperature. It makes a stunning centerpiece for summer gatherings or a special treat for family desserts.

Autumn Root Vegetable Roast with Herbs

Autumn Root Vegetable Roast with Herbs is a comforting and nourishing dish that highlights the hearty flavors of seasonal root vegetables and aromatic herbs. Autumn is the time when root vegetables such as carrots, parsnips, sweet potatoes, and turnips are at their peak, offering a rich source of vitamins, minerals, and fiber. Roasting these vegetables enhances their natural sweetness and caramelizes their edges, while fresh herbs such as rosemary, thyme, and sage add depth and aroma to the dish.

To prepare Autumn Root Vegetable Roast with Herbs, start by selecting a variety of root vegetables in different colors and textures. Peel and cut the vegetables into uniform pieces to ensure even cooking. Toss the vegetables in a bowl with olive oil, minced garlic, chopped fresh herbs (such as rosemary, thyme, and sage), sea salt, and freshly ground black pepper.

Spread the seasoned vegetables in a single layer on a baking sheet lined with parchment paper or a silicone baking mat. Roast in a preheated oven at 400°F (200°C) for 30-40 minutes, or until the vegetables are tender and caramelized, stirring halfway through cooking to ensure even browning.

Once roasted, transfer the vegetables to a serving dish and garnish with additional fresh herbs for a pop of color and flavor. Autumn Root Vegetable Roast with Herbs can be served as a hearty side dish alongside roasted meats or poultry, or as a vegetarian main course with a grain or salad.

Winter Squash Soup with Nutmeg and Cinnamon

Winter Squash Soup with Nutmeg and Cinnamon is a comforting and warming dish that captures the essence of winter with its rich, velvety texture and aromatic spices. Winter squash varieties such as butternut squash, acorn squash, or pumpkin are naturally sweet and creamy when cooked, making them ideal for soups. Nutmeg and cinnamon add a warm, spicy flavor that complements the sweetness of the squash, creating a soup that is both comforting and satisfying on cold winter days.

To prepare Winter Squash Soup with Nutmeg and Cinnamon, start by selecting a winter squash such as butternut squash or pumpkin. Peel and cut the squash into cubes, discarding the seeds and fibrous pulp. You can also roast the squash halves in the oven until tender and scoop out the flesh for added depth of flavor.

In a large pot, heat olive oil or butter over medium heat. Add diced onions and minced garlic, cooking until softened and fragrant. Add the cubed squash to the pot along with vegetable broth, water, or coconut milk for a creamy texture. Season with ground nutmeg, cinnamon, sea salt, and freshly ground black pepper to taste.

Simmer the soup over medium-low heat for 20-25 minutes, or until the squash is tender and easily mashed with a fork. Use an immersion blender to puree the soup until smooth and creamy. Alternatively, you can transfer the soup in batches to a blender and blend until smooth, taking care not to overfill the blender with hot liquid.

Once blended, return the soup to the pot and adjust the seasoning to taste. If desired, stir in a splash of coconut milk or cream for added richness. Serve the Winter Squash Soup with Nutmeg and Cinnamon hot, garnished with a sprinkle of fresh herbs such as parsley or a dollop of plain yogurt.

This soup is perfect for warming up on chilly winter evenings and can be served as a comforting appetizer or a light main course with crusty bread or a side salad. Its creamy texture and aromatic spices make it a favorite among both adults and children alike during the colder months.

In summary, each of these seasonal recipes celebrates the flavors and ingredients of its respective season, offering both nourishment and enjoyment. From the fresh, vibrant flavors of the Spring Foraged Salad with Violets and Sorrel to the comforting warmth of the Winter Squash Soup with Nutmeg and Cinnamon, these recipes showcase the best of seasonal eating and highlight the natural bounty that each season has to offer. Whether you're looking for a light and refreshing salad, a decadent dessert, a hearty vegetable dish, or a comforting soup, these recipes are sure to delight your senses and nourish your body throughout the year.

Chapter 21: Special Diets from Historical Contexts

Dairy-Free Almond Milk Pottage

Dairy-Free Almond Milk Pottage is a historical dish that dates back to medieval times when dairy alternatives were often used due to dietary restrictions or availability. Pottage itself refers to a thick soup or stew made with vegetables, grains, and sometimes meat, often cooked slowly to create a hearty and nutritious meal. Almond milk, made by blending almonds with water and straining the mixture, serves as a creamy base in this version, replacing traditional dairy milk.

To prepare Dairy-Free Almond Milk Pottage, start by soaking raw almonds in water overnight or for at least a few hours. Drain and rinse the almonds, then blend them with fresh water until smooth. Strain the almond mixture through a cheesecloth or nut milk bag to extract the milk, squeezing out as much liquid as possible. The resulting almond milk will be creamy and slightly nutty in flavor, perfect for cooking and baking.

In a large pot, heat olive oil or butter over medium heat. Add diced onions, garlic, and chopped vegetables such as carrots, celery, and leeks. Sauté until the vegetables are softened and fragrant. Add grains such as barley, oats, or quinoa, stirring to coat with the vegetables and oil.

Pour in the almond milk and vegetable broth, bringing the mixture to a simmer. Season with salt, pepper, and herbs such as thyme, rosemary, or sage, adjusting the flavors to taste. Simmer the pottage over low heat, stirring occasionally, until the grains are cooked through and the mixture has thickened to a stew-like consistency.

Serve Dairy-Free Almond Milk Pottage hot, garnished with fresh herbs or a drizzle of olive oil. This hearty dish provides a comforting meal that is both dairy-free and rich in plant-based protein, fiber, and essential nutrients.

Paleo Bison Stew with Marrow Bones

Paleo Bison Stew with Marrow Bones is inspired by the ancestral diet of Paleolithic humans who relied on wild game, nuts, seeds, fruits, and vegetables. Bison, a lean and nutrient-dense meat, is rich in protein, iron, and essential amino acids, making it an excellent choice for a Paleo-inspired stew. Marrow bones, prized for their rich, buttery marrow, add depth of flavor and provide beneficial nutrients such as vitamins A and K2, omega-3 fatty acids, and collagen.

To prepare Paleo Bison Stew with Marrow Bones, start by browning bison stew meat in a large pot with olive oil or ghee over medium-high heat. Once the meat is browned on all sides, remove it from the pot and set it aside. Add diced onions, garlic, and chopped vegetables such as carrots, celery, and bell peppers to the pot, sautéing until softened and aromatic.

Return the browned bison meat to the pot, along with beef or bison bone broth to cover the ingredients. Add herbs such as bay leaves, thyme, and oregano for flavor, and season with sea salt and freshly ground black pepper to taste. Bring the stew to a boil, then reduce the heat to low and simmer gently for 2-3 hours, or until the meat is tender and falls apart easily.

During the last hour of cooking, add marrow bones to the stew, nestling them among the meat and vegetables. The marrow bones will release their rich, nutrient-dense marrow into the stew, adding depth and richness to the broth.

Serve Paleo Bison Stew with Marrow Bones hot, garnished with fresh herbs such as parsley or chives. This hearty stew provides a satisfying and nourishing meal that adheres to Paleo principles while celebrating the flavors and benefits of wild game and bone marrow.

Vegan Roasted Vegetable and Nut Loaf

Vegan Roasted Vegetable and Nut Loaf is a plant-based twist on the classic meatloaf, offering a hearty and satisfying dish that is packed with vegetables, nuts, seeds, and savory herbs. This loaf is perfect for vegans or anyone looking to incorporate more plant-based meals into their diet without sacrificing flavor or texture. Roasted vegetables such as sweet potatoes, bell peppers, zucchini, and mushrooms provide a hearty base, while nuts and seeds add protein, healthy fats, and crunch.

To prepare Vegan Roasted Vegetable and Nut Loaf, start by roasting a variety of vegetables in the oven until tender and caramelized. You can toss the vegetables with olive oil, garlic, and herbs such as thyme or rosemary before roasting to enhance their flavor. Once roasted, let the vegetables cool slightly, then chop them into small pieces.

In a large mixing bowl, combine the roasted vegetables with cooked quinoa or brown rice for added texture and nutrition. Add a mixture of finely chopped nuts and seeds such as walnuts, almonds, sunflower seeds, and flaxseeds for protein and healthy fats. Season the mixture with soy sauce or tamari, nutritional yeast, and herbs such as parsley or sage for savory flavor.

Transfer the vegetable and nut mixture to a loaf pan lined with parchment paper, pressing it down firmly to mold into a loaf shape. Bake the loaf in a preheated oven at 350°F (175°C) for 45-50 minutes, or until the top is golden brown and the loaf is firm to the touch.

Let the Vegan Roasted Vegetable and Nut Loaf cool in the pan for 10-15 minutes before slicing and serving. This loaf can be enjoyed hot or cold and makes a delicious main course or hearty sandwich filling. Serve it with a side of steamed vegetables or a fresh green salad for a complete and balanced meal.

In conclusion, these special diet recipes from historical contexts offer a glimpse into traditional and ancestral ways of eating that prioritize nutrient-dense ingredients and whole foods. From the dairy-free innovation of Almond Milk Pottage to the Paleo-inspired richness of Bison Stew with Marrow Bones and the plant-based creativity of Vegan Roasted Vegetable and Nut Loaf, each dish celebrates the diversity and benefits of different dietary approaches while providing delicious and satisfying meals for modern palates.

Chapter 22: Rediscovered Cooking Techniques

Open Hearth Cooking Methods

Open hearth cooking, a time-honored tradition, connects us to the culinary practices of our ancestors. This method of cooking involves the use of a large open fireplace, often equipped with iron hardware, where various types of food are cooked over an open flame or hot coals. The open hearth kitchen was once the heart of the home, providing warmth and a place to prepare meals.

The techniques of open hearth cooking are diverse and require skill and patience. One primary method is roasting. Traditionally, meats are cooked on a spit, a long metal rod that can be turned to ensure even cooking. The meat is placed on the spit and positioned over the fire. Turning the spit manually or with the aid of a mechanical spit jack ensures that the meat cooks evenly and maintains its juices. This method is particularly effective for larger cuts of meat such as whole chickens, turkeys, or large roasts.

Baking in an open hearth typically involves the use of Dutch ovens, heavy cast iron pots with tight-fitting lids. These versatile cooking vessels can be placed directly in the coals or suspended above the fire. The Dutch oven can bake bread, pies, and even casseroles. When baking bread, coals are often placed on top of the lid as well as underneath the pot to create an even cooking environment similar to a modern oven.

Boiling and stewing are also integral to open hearth cooking. Large pots or kettles are suspended over the fire using a crane, an adjustable arm that swings in and out of the heat. This setup allows for precise temperature control, as the pot can be moved closer to or farther from the flames. Stews, soups, and boiled dishes can simmer slowly, developing rich flavors over time.

Another fascinating method is plank cooking. In this technique, fish or other meats are placed on wooden planks and set near the fire. The heat from the fire cooks the food while the wood imparts a subtle flavor. Cedar planks are particularly popular for this method due to their aromatic qualities.

The use of hot stones is an ancient technique still employed in open hearth cooking. Stones are heated in the fire and then used to cook food either directly on the stones or by placing them in a pit or container with the food. This method is excellent for cooking items like flatbreads or even for steaming food wrapped in leaves.

Grilling is a straightforward and popular method in open hearth cooking. Foods are placed on a grill rack over the fire, similar to modern barbecue methods. This technique works well for meats, vegetables, and even fruits. The open flame imparts a unique flavor that is difficult to replicate with other cooking methods.

Beyond these primary techniques, open hearth cooking also encompasses methods like ember roasting and ash baking. Ember roasting involves cooking food directly in the hot embers of the fire. This method is ideal for root vegetables like potatoes or beets, which develop a smoky flavor and tender texture. Ash baking, on the other hand, involves burying food in the ashes of the fire to cook slowly. This method is traditionally used for items like sweet potatoes or bread wrapped in leaves or dough.

Safety and efficiency are crucial considerations in open hearth cooking. Properly maintaining the fire, using the right tools, and understanding how to control the heat are essential skills. Modern enthusiasts of open hearth cooking often rely on historical texts and reenactments to learn these skills, preserving the knowledge for future generations.

Open hearth cooking is more than just a way to prepare food; it is a connection to the past, a way to experience the flavors and techniques of our ancestors. The methods used in open hearth cooking can bring a new depth of flavor and a sense of history to the food we eat today.

Salt Curing and Smoking of Meats

Salt curing and smoking are ancient preservation techniques that have been used for centuries to extend the shelf life of meats and impart distinctive flavors. These methods, once essential for survival, have evolved into cherished culinary arts that continue to captivate food enthusiasts.

Salt curing, one of the oldest preservation methods, involves the use of salt to draw moisture out of the meat, creating an environment inhospitable to bacteria. There are several types of salt curing, each with its unique characteristics and uses. Dry curing is the most straightforward method, where the meat is rubbed with a mixture of salt, sugar, and spices. The meat is then stored in a cool, dry place for several weeks. This method is commonly used for hams, bacon, and some sausages.

Wet curing, also known as brining, involves immersing the meat in a solution of salt, water, and other seasonings. The meat absorbs the brine, which helps to preserve it and add flavor. This method is often used for poultry and pork. The brine can be infused with various herbs, spices, and even sweeteners like molasses or honey to create a complex flavor profile.

Equilibrium curing is a modern approach to salt curing, offering more precise control over the salt content. In this method, a calculated amount of salt is used based on the weight of the meat, ensuring that the final product is perfectly seasoned without being overly salty. This method is particularly useful for those looking to create consistent results and avoid the guesswork often associated with traditional curing methods.

Smoking, another time-honored preservation technique, involves exposing the meat to smoke from burning wood. This process not only preserves the meat but also imparts a rich, smoky flavor that is highly prized in many culinary traditions. There are two primary types of smoking: cold smoking and hot smoking.

Cold smoking is a method where the meat is exposed to smoke at a low temperature, typically below 90°F (32°C). This process can take several days to weeks, depending on the size and type of meat. Cold smoking does not cook the meat but rather infuses it with smoke flavor while continuing the curing process. This method is commonly used for products like smoked salmon, jerky, and certain types of sausages.

Hot smoking, on the other hand, involves cooking the meat while it is being smoked. The temperature in the smoking chamber is maintained between 165°F (74°C) and 250°F

(121°C), effectively cooking the meat and infusing it with smoke flavor. This method is faster than cold smoking and results in ready-to-eat products like smoked brisket, ribs, and poultry.

The choice of wood is a critical factor in smoking, as different woods impart different flavors. Hardwoods like oak, hickory, and maple are popular choices, each providing a unique flavor profile. Fruitwoods like apple, cherry, and peach offer a milder, sweeter smoke, ideal for poultry and fish. Experimenting with different wood combinations can yield a wide range of flavors, allowing for endless culinary creativity.

The combination of salt curing and smoking can produce some of the most celebrated meat products in the culinary world. Prosciutto, a dry-cured Italian ham, undergoes a lengthy curing process followed by months of air drying. The result is a delicately flavored, melt-in-your-mouth delicacy. Smoked bacon, another beloved product, begins with a salt cure before being hot smoked to perfection.

Safety is a paramount consideration in salt curing and smoking. Proper sanitation, temperature control, and the use of curing salts containing nitrates or nitrites help prevent the growth of harmful bacteria such as Clostridium botulinum. These curing agents also contribute to the characteristic color and flavor of cured meats.

Salt curing and smoking are more than just preservation methods; they are culinary arts that require patience, precision, and a deep understanding of the processes involved. These techniques allow us to transform simple cuts of meat into complex, flavorful delicacies that connect us to the culinary traditions of the past.

Solar Drying of Fruits and Herbs

Solar drying, an ancient method of preserving fruits and herbs, harnesses the power of the sun to remove moisture from food, extending its shelf life and concentrating its flavors. This technique, deeply rooted in tradition, is both environmentally friendly and accessible, making it a valuable skill for modern home cooks and gardeners.

The process of solar drying is straightforward but requires careful attention to detail to ensure optimal results. The first step is selecting the right fruits and herbs. For fruits, it is essential to choose ripe, unblemished produce. Commonly dried fruits include apples, apricots, berries, grapes (for raisins), and plums (for prunes). Herbs suitable for drying include basil, oregano, rosemary, thyme, mint, and sage. Harvesting herbs at their peak, just before flowering, ensures maximum flavor retention.

Preparation of fruits for solar drying typically involves washing, peeling, and slicing the produce into uniform pieces. Smaller pieces dry more quickly and evenly, reducing the risk of spoilage. Some fruits, such as apples and pears, benefit from a brief dip in a solution of lemon juice and water to prevent browning. For herbs, simply rinse them under cool water and pat dry with a clean towel.

The drying setup can vary, but a basic solar dryer consists of a wooden frame covered with fine mesh or cheesecloth. This structure allows air to circulate around the food while protecting it from insects and debris. Alternatively, commercially available solar dehydrators provide more controlled environments and often feature adjustable trays and vents for better airflow.

Positioning the solar dryer is critical for efficient drying. It should be placed in a sunny, well-ventilated area, ideally elevated off the ground to maximize air circulation. The drying process can take several days, depending on the humidity, temperature, and type of food being dried. Turning the food periodically ensures even drying and prevents sticking.

For fruits, the drying time varies based on the type and thickness of the slices. Apples and pears may take 2-3 days, while berries can take up to a week. The fruit is considered adequately dried when it feels leathery and no longer releases moisture when pressed. Herbs dry more quickly, usually within 1-3 days. Properly dried herbs should crumble easily between your fingers

and retain their vibrant color and aroma.

Storage is the final step in the solar drying process. Once fully dried, fruits should be cooled to room temperature and stored in airtight containers or resealable bags. Properly dried fruits can be stored for several months to a year in a cool, dark place. Herbs should be stored whole in airtight containers away from light and heat to preserve their flavor and potency.

Solar drying offers numerous benefits beyond preservation. It enhances the flavor of fruits and herbs by concentrating their natural sugars and essential oils. Dried fruits make nutritious snacks or additions to cereals, baked goods, and trail mixes. Dried herbs can elevate culinary dishes, infuse oils and vinegars, or be brewed into teas for their medicinal properties.

From an environmental standpoint, solar drying is energy-efficient and reduces reliance on electricity or fossil fuels. By utilizing renewable solar energy, home cooks can embrace sustainable food preservation practices that minimize their carbon footprint.

In conclusion, solar drying is a time-tested method that allows home cooks and gardeners to preserve the bounty of the harvest while enhancing flavors and promoting sustainability. Whether drying fruits for sweet treats or herbs for culinary creations, mastering the art of solar drying connects us to our agricultural heritage and ensures delicious, nutrient-rich foods year-round.

Chapter 23: Superfoods of the Ancients

Spirulina and Barley Flatbreads

Spirulina, a blue-green algae packed with nutrients, has been consumed for centuries by various cultures around the world. Its rich protein content, abundance of vitamins and minerals, and antioxidant properties make it a prized superfood. Combined with barley, an ancient grain known for its nutty flavor and nutritional benefits, spirulina transforms into a versatile ingredient for flatbreads.

To prepare spirulina and barley flatbreads, start by mixing whole barley flour with water to form a dough. Incorporate powdered spirulina into the dough, kneading it thoroughly to distribute the algae evenly. Spirulina not only adds a vibrant green color to the dough but also boosts its nutritional profile with essential amino acids, vitamins (like B12), and iron.

Once the dough is well-mixed, divide it into portions and roll each portion into thin rounds. Traditionally, these flatbreads are cooked on a hot griddle or skillet until they develop a golden-brown color and slightly crispy texture. The flatbreads can be enjoyed warm with toppings like hummus, fresh vegetables, or as a side to soups and stews.

The combination of spirulina and barley not only creates a visually striking dish but also offers a complete source of plant-based protein, essential fatty acids, and fiber. This nutrient-dense flatbread is an excellent addition to a balanced diet, providing sustained energy and supporting overall health.

Hemp Seed and Wild Honey Porridge

Hemp seeds, derived from the Cannabis sativa plant, are a nutritional powerhouse rich in omega-3 and omega-6 fatty acids, protein, and various vitamins and minerals. Combined with wild honey, a natural sweetener revered since ancient times for its flavor and medicinal properties, hemp seeds create a nourishing porridge that satisfies both the palate and nutritional needs.

To prepare hemp seed and wild honey porridge, start by simmering hemp seeds in water or milk (dairy or plant-based) until they soften and absorb the liquid. The hemp seeds release a creamy texture as they cook, similar to traditional porridge grains like oats or quinoa. Stirring occasionally prevents sticking and ensures even cooking.

Once the hemp seeds reach a porridge-like consistency, sweeten the mixture with wild honey to taste. Wild honey, sourced from bees that forage on wildflowers, offers a distinct floral flavor and potential health benefits due to its natural enzymes and antioxidants. Stir the honey into the porridge until well incorporated.

Serve the hemp seed and wild honey porridge warm, optionally garnished with fresh fruits, nuts, or seeds for added texture and flavor. This hearty dish is not only comforting but also provides a balanced blend of carbohydrates, healthy fats, and protein. It makes an ideal breakfast option or wholesome snack for sustained energy throughout the day.

Chia and Acai Berry Pudding

Chia seeds, known for their high fiber content and omega-3 fatty acids, were a staple food of ancient Mesoamerican civilizations like the Aztecs and Mayans. Acai berries, native to the Amazon rainforest and revered for their antioxidant properties and rich purple color, complement chia seeds in a decadent pudding that celebrates both taste and health benefits.

To prepare chia and acai berry pudding, begin by soaking chia seeds in a liquid such as coconut milk or almond milk. The chia seeds absorb the liquid and swell, creating a gel-like consistency that forms the base of the pudding. Allow the mixture to rest for at least 30 minutes or refrigerate overnight to achieve a thicker texture.

Meanwhile, prepare the acai berry component by blending frozen acai berries with a small amount of liquid until smooth. Acai berries are perishable and typically sold in freeze-dried or frozen form to preserve their nutrients. The vibrant purple hue of acai berries adds a visually appealing contrast to the chia seed pudding.

To assemble the pudding, layer the soaked chia seeds with the blended acai berry mixture in serving cups or bowls. Alternate layers for a visually striking presentation and a harmonious blend of flavors. Chill the pudding in the refrigerator for a few hours to allow the flavors to meld and the pudding to set further.

Chia and acai berry pudding is a delightful dessert or snack option that combines the nutritional benefits of both superfoods. It is naturally sweetened and loaded with antioxidants, fiber, and essential nutrients. Enjoy this pudding chilled, garnished with fresh berries, shredded coconut, or a drizzle of honey for added sweetness.

In conclusion, incorporating superfoods like spirulina, hemp seeds, chia seeds, and acai berries into everyday meals connects us to ancient culinary traditions while providing modern health benefits. These nutrient-dense ingredients offer a wealth of vitamins, minerals, and antioxidants that support overall well-being and contribute to a diverse and flavorful diet.

Chapter 24: Mindful Eating Practices from the Past

Rituals Around Meals

Rituals around meals have been an integral part of human culture since ancient times, serving not only to nourish the body but also to foster social bonds, express gratitude, and honor traditions. Across different civilizations and eras, mealtime rituals vary widely but share a common thread of mindfulness and reverence for food.

In ancient Greece, for example, communal feasting was a significant social event where friends and family gathered to share food and conversation. The symposium, a formal banquet, was a platform for philosophical discussions and artistic performances, emphasizing the connection between food, intellect, and community.

In traditional Japanese culture, the tea ceremony (chanoyu) is a profound ritual centered around the preparation and consumption of matcha tea. Practiced for centuries, the tea ceremony embodies principles of harmony, respect, purity, and tranquility (wa, kei, sei, jaku). Participants engage in deliberate movements and gestures, savoring each moment as they prepare and enjoy the tea.

Among Indigenous peoples around the world, mealtime rituals often involve prayers, songs, and storytelling to honor the Earth and the spirits that sustain life. Food is viewed as a gift from the land and the ancestors, reinforcing a spiritual connection to nature and a deep sense of gratitude for the bounty provided.

Modern mindfulness practices draw inspiration from these ancient mealtime rituals, encouraging individuals to slow down, savor each bite, and cultivate gratitude for the nourishment received. By adopting rituals around meals, we can enhance our appreciation for food, strengthen social bonds, and promote holistic well-being.

The Importance of Eating Seasonally and Locally

Eating seasonally and locally is a practice rooted in ancient wisdom that aligns food consumption with natural cycles and local ecosystems. Before the advent of global food transportation, people relied on foods that were abundant and ripe during specific seasons, optimizing nutritional intake and flavor variety.

Seasonal eating encourages a diverse and nutrient-rich diet. Spring brings tender greens, fresh herbs, and early fruits like strawberries and asparagus, rich in vitamins and antioxidants to rejuvenate after winter. Summer offers an abundance of vibrant vegetables, berries, and stone fruits, providing hydration and energy during warmer months.

Autumn harvests yield hearty root vegetables, pumpkins, apples, and nuts, packed with vitamins, fiber, and complex carbohydrates to support immunity and warmth as temperatures cool. Winter brings citrus fruits, cruciferous vegetables, and storage crops like squash and potatoes, rich in vitamin C and essential nutrients to bolster resilience against seasonal illnesses.

Eating locally supports community agriculture and reduces the environmental impact of food production and transportation. Farmers' markets, community-supported agriculture (CSA) programs, and garden harvests reconnect consumers with the origins of their food, fostering appreciation for local growers and seasonal bounty.

Adopting a seasonal and local eating approach promotes sustainability, reduces food miles, and celebrates regional culinary traditions. It encourages flexibility and creativity in meal planning while maximizing nutritional benefits and supporting environmental stewardship.

Mindfulness in Preparation and Consumption

Mindfulness in food preparation and consumption involves conscious awareness and intentional focus on the sensory experience of eating. Ancient cultures recognized the transformative power of mindful eating practices to enhance digestion, promote satiety, and cultivate gratitude for food as nourishment.

In Ayurveda, the traditional healing system of India, mindful eating is a cornerstone of health and well-being. Ayurvedic principles emphasize eating in a calm, peaceful environment, free from distractions, to enhance digestion and absorption of nutrients. Foods are chosen and prepared mindfully according to one's unique constitution (dosha) and seasonal influences.

In traditional Chinese medicine (TCM), mindful eating practices are rooted in the concept of food energetics and the balance of yin and yang energies. Meals are prepared with attention to color, flavor, texture, and temperature to harmonize internal energies and support optimal health. Chewed slowly and thoroughly, food is savored to aid digestion and promote nutrient assimilation.

The practice of mindfulness in food preparation involves mindful ingredient selection, thoughtful cooking techniques, and appreciation for the transformation of raw ingredients into nourishing meals. Cooking becomes a meditative practice, enhancing culinary skills and fostering creativity in the kitchen.

Mindfulness in food consumption extends beyond the act of eating to include mindful portion sizes, chewing slowly, and tuning into hunger and satiety cues. By eating mindfully, we can develop a deeper connection to our bodies' nutritional needs, reduce overeating, and cultivate a more balanced relationship with food.

In conclusion, mindful eating practices from the past offer valuable insights into fostering gratitude, enhancing nutritional intake, and promoting overall well-being. By embracing mealtime rituals, eating seasonally and locally, and cultivating mindfulness in food preparation and consumption, we can reconnect with ancient wisdom and cultivate healthier, more fulfilling relationships with food and ourselves.

Chapter 25: Reconnecting With Nature Through Food

Edible Wild Plant Identification and Use

Edible wild plants offer a unique opportunity to reconnect with nature and enhance our diet with nutritious, natural foods. Identifying and using these plants require knowledge and practice but can lead to a rewarding and sustainable lifestyle. One must start by familiarizing themselves with common edible wild plants in their region. Local field guides, plant identification apps, and foraging workshops can be invaluable resources. When identifying plants, focus on key features such as leaves, stems, flowers, and fruits. Pay attention to the plant's habitat, as certain plants thrive in specific environments like woodlands, meadows, or wetlands.

Safety is paramount when foraging. Always ensure positive identification before consuming any wild plant, as some edible plants have toxic look-alikes. For example, wild carrots can be mistaken for poison hemlock, which is deadly. Consulting multiple sources and experts can help prevent such mistakes. Additionally, start by trying small quantities of new plants to rule out any allergies or adverse reactions.

Once identified, understanding the uses of these plants is essential. Many wild plants are rich in vitamins, minerals, and antioxidants, often surpassing their cultivated counterparts in nutritional value. For instance, dandelion greens are high in vitamins A, C, and K, and their roots can be used to make a caffeine-free coffee substitute. Stinging nettle, despite its name, loses its sting when cooked and is a great source of iron and protein.

Preparing wild plants can be as simple as adding them to salads, soups, or teas. Some, like purslane, can be eaten raw and have a slightly tangy, lemony flavor, while others, such as burdock root, are better cooked. Experimenting with different recipes can help integrate these plants into everyday meals.

Beyond nutrition, foraging for wild plants can have therapeutic benefits. It encourages physical activity, mindfulness, and a deeper connection to the natural world. By observing the seasons and local ecosystems, foragers develop a greater appreciation for the environment and its cycles.

Incorporating wild plants into one's diet not only diversifies nutrition but also promotes sustainability. Wild plants require no cultivation, fertilizers, or pesticides, making them an eco-friendly food source. Moreover, foraging can reduce food costs and dependency on commercial agriculture, which often has significant environmental impacts.

However, responsible foraging is crucial. Always harvest sustainably by taking only what is needed and leaving enough for the plant to reproduce and support wildlife. Avoid overharvesting in any given area to prevent depletion of resources. Additionally, respect private property and obtain necessary permissions before foraging on non-public land.

Creating a Kitchen Garden with Heirloom Plants

Creating a kitchen garden with heirloom plants is a delightful way to reconnect with nature and enjoy a diverse array of flavors, textures, and colors in your meals. Heirloom plants, which are open-pollinated and passed down through generations, offer genetic diversity and superior taste compared to many modern hybrids. Starting a kitchen garden involves careful planning, preparation, and maintenance, but the rewards are well worth the effort.

Begin by selecting an appropriate location for your garden. Most heirloom plants thrive in full sun, requiring at least six to eight hours of direct sunlight daily. The chosen site should have well-drained soil and easy access to water. Raised beds or container gardening can be excellent options for those with limited space or poor soil quality.

Preparing the soil is a crucial step. Test the soil's pH and nutrient levels to determine any necessary amendments. Heirloom plants generally prefer soil that is rich in organic matter. Incorporate compost or well-rotted manure to improve soil fertility and structure. This will create an ideal environment for seed germination and root development.

Choosing heirloom varieties is one of the most exciting aspects of creating a kitchen garden. Heirloom seeds are often available from specialized seed companies, local farmers' markets, and seed exchanges. Consider selecting a diverse range of vegetables, herbs, and flowers that suit your climate and growing conditions. For example, heirloom tomatoes come in a rainbow of colors and flavors, from the sweet and juicy Brandywine to the rich and tangy Cherokee Purple. Heirloom beans, such as the speckled Jacob's Cattle or the buttery Christmas Lima, add variety to your diet and garden.

Planting heirloom seeds involves following specific guidelines for each type of plant. Some seeds, like tomatoes and peppers, benefit from being started indoors several weeks before the last frost date. Others, such as beans and squash, can be sown directly into the garden once the soil has warmed. Follow the recommended spacing and planting depth for each seed variety to ensure optimal growth.

Regular watering and mulching are essential for maintaining a healthy kitchen garden. Heirloom plants often require consistent moisture but do not tolerate waterlogged soil. Mulching with organic materials like straw or wood chips helps retain soil moisture, suppress weeds, and regulate soil temperature. Additionally, practicing crop rotation and companion planting can help manage pests and diseases naturally.

Heirloom plants often have unique growth habits and care requirements. For example, some heirloom tomatoes may require staking or caging to support their heavy fruit loads, while heirloom lettuces might bolt quickly in hot weather and benefit from shade cloth. Paying attention to these details can enhance your gardening success.

Harvesting heirloom produce at its peak ripeness ensures the best flavor and nutritional value. Many heirloom vegetables, such as tomatoes and peppers, should be picked when fully ripe and colored. Others, like beans and peas, are best harvested when young and tender. Regular harvesting encourages continuous production and prevents overripening.

Preserving heirloom seeds from your garden is a rewarding practice that promotes sustainability and self-sufficiency. Allow some of your healthiest plants to go to seed, and then collect and store the seeds for future planting. Properly dried and stored seeds can remain viable for several years, ensuring a continuous supply of heirloom varieties.

Creating a kitchen garden with heirloom plants is more than just growing food; it's about preserving biodiversity, honoring agricultural heritage, and enjoying the profound connection to nature that comes from tending the land. Each heirloom plant has a story, a history that enriches the gardening experience and the meals you prepare from your harvest.

Foraging Techniques and Seasonal Harvests

Foraging for wild food is an ancient practice that connects us to the rhythms of nature and the bounty of our local ecosystems. Understanding foraging techniques and the seasonality of wild plants can transform your approach to food, making each meal a testament to the natural world's abundance.

Successful foraging begins with education and preparation. Equip yourself with the right tools, including a good-quality foraging knife, a basket or cloth bag for collecting plants, and a field guide for plant identification. Dress appropriately for the terrain and weather, and always inform someone of your foraging plans and expected return time.

Seasonal knowledge is crucial in foraging. Different plants are available at different times of the year, each season offering its unique treasures. Spring is a prime time for tender greens and wildflowers, such as ramps, chickweed, and violets. These early plants are often rich in vitamins and can invigorate the diet after a long winter.

Summer brings a wealth of fruits, berries, and herbs. Blackberries, raspberries, and elderberries are ripe for the picking, while aromatic herbs like mint and yarrow are at their peak. This season is ideal for gathering ingredients for jams, teas, and fresh salads.

Autumn is the time to harvest nuts, roots, and late-season fruits. Acorns, chestnuts, and walnuts can be foraged and processed into nutritious flours and butters. Roots like burdock and wild carrots are best dug up before the ground freezes, providing hearty additions to soups and stews.

Winter foraging is more challenging but not impossible. Some greens, like chickweed and miner's lettuce, can survive mild winters. Additionally, pine needles and certain tree barks can be harvested for teas and medicinal uses.

Foraging techniques vary depending on the plant and its habitat. Here are some general guidelines:

1. **Leaves and Greens**: When foraging for greens, such as dandelion or nettle, use a sharp knife or scissors to cut the leaves at the base, leaving the root intact to encourage regrowth. Harvest young, tender leaves for the best flavor and nutritional value.

2. **Fruits and Berries**: Pick fruits and berries gently to avoid damaging the plant. Use a basket to prevent squashing delicate berries. Only take what you need and leave enough for wildlife and plant reproduction.

3. **Roots and Tubers**: Use a digging stick or trowel to carefully unearth roots and tubers. Be mindful of the plant's role in the ecosystem and harvest sparingly. Clean roots thoroughly and remove any fibrous or woody parts.

4. **Seeds and Nuts**: Collect seeds and nuts by hand, shaking or gently stripping them from the plant. Some nuts, like acorns, require leaching to remove tannins before consumption.

5. **Mushrooms**: Foraging for mushrooms requires expertise due to the presence of toxic species. Use a knife to cut mushrooms at the base and carry them in a mesh bag to allow spore dispersal. Only harvest mushrooms that you can positively identify as edible.

Ethical foraging practices are essential to preserve the environment and ensure sustainable harvests. Never overharvest a single area or deplete a plant population. Take only what you need and leave enough for the plant to thrive and reproduce. Avoid foraging in protected areas or private property without permission.

Respecting nature's balance and understanding your role in the ecosystem is fundamental. Foraging provides an opportunity to observe and learn from nature, deepening your connection to the land. This mindful approach can transform foraging from a simple act of gathering food into a profound experience of ecological stewardship and appreciation.

Foraging not only diversifies your diet with wild, nutrient-dense

foods but also reconnects you to ancestral practices and seasonal rhythms. By embracing foraging techniques and understanding seasonal harvests, you embark on a journey of discovery and sustainability, where each foraged ingredient tells a story of resilience and adaptation in the natural world.

THE END

Made in United States
Orlando, FL
04 October 2024